PSYCHIATRIC ONCOLOGY

Critical Essays in the Psychosocial Spectrum of Cancer Care

by John H. Morgan

PSYCHIATRIC ONCOLOGY

Critical Essays in the Psychosocial Spectrum of Cancer Care

John H. Morgan

Ph.D.(Hartford), D.Sc.(London), Psy.D.(FH/Oxford)

Senior Fellow in Behavioral Science *emeritus*

Foundation House/Oxford (UK)

978-155605-536-2 Paperback

978-155605-537-9 E Book

Wyndham Hall Press

N. Fort Myers, FL

ACKNOWLEDGEMENTS 7

INTRODUCTION

A SPECIALIZATION IN CANCER CARE AND TREATMENT 9

CHAPTER ONE

EMOTIONAL CARE AND TREATMENT OF THE CANCER PATIENT: The Oncology Specialization addressing the Psychosocial Dynamics of Healing ...12

CHAPTER TWO

THE LABELING OF PSYCHIATRIC ONCOLOGY: Its Meaning and Development 28

CHAPTER THREE

THE SCOPE OF DESCRIPTIVE PSYCHIATRY (Emil Kraepelin, M.D., in profile).......................34

CHAPTER FOUR

THE SCOPE OF INTERPERSONAL PSYCHIATRY (Harry Stack Sullivan, M.D., in profile) 49

CHAPTER FIVE

THE EMOTIONAL SPECTRUM OF A TERMINAL DIAGNOSIS: Addressing the Psychosocial Issues in Psychiatric Oncology 69

CHAPTER SIX

A RANGE OF SPECIALIZED PROGRAMS IN PSYCHIATRIC ONCOLOGY: Leading Medical Institutions in the United States 84

CHAPTER SEVEN

A CROSS-CULTURAL APPROACH TO PSYCHIATRIC ONCOLOGY: Consultation Liaison Psychiatry in Clinical Profile 106

CHAPTER EIGHT

PSYCHIATRIC ONCOLOGY IN REVIEW: Two Decades and More of Pivotal Research 126

APPENDICES

A. RELIGIOUS FAITH AND SCIENTIFIC ACCOUNTABILITY: Exploring the False Conundrum in Medical Oncology 152

B. MEDICATION AND COUNSELING IN PSYCHIATRIC PRACTICE: Biogenic Psychopharmacology and Psychogenic Psychotherapy 157

C. JIMMIE C. HOLLAND, M.D. 160

BIBLIOGRAPHICAL REFERENCES AND RESOURCES 161

BOOKS BY JOHN H. MORGAN 190

ABOUT THE AUTHOR 192

ACKNOWLEDGEMENTS

The background to the development of this book has a long history but the writing of it has been quite short. I first became interested in the relationship between the practice of medicine and society when I taught a course on the subject early in my career at the University of Connecticut. I continued my interest during my six years of postdoctoral fellowships in the behavioral sciences at Harvard, Yale, and Princeton when I published my first book on the subject titled *Third World Medicine and Social Change.* The maturing of my interest commenced during my twenty years of teaching a doctoral-level seminar in the International Summer Programme of Oxford University while being the Editor of a scholarly periodical, *The Behavioral Mind: A Journal of Personality Disorders.* However, I decided to take up a serious address to the issues involved in psychiatric oncology following a conversation with my oncologist, Rashid Khan, M.D., resulting from a diagnosis of cancer which I have been battling for the past five years.

This book is essentially a product of all of these experiences coalescing into a collection of critical essays dealing with some of the key topics involved in the treatment of cancer patients. The point of view of the psychosocial spectrum of cancer care is here perceived as offering a balanced treatment plan to the bio-medical side of patient care. I owe deep gratitude to a plethora of scholars and professional practitioners linked to the outstanding institutions with which I have been privileged to be affiliated with in my long teaching and research career. Finally, to my family who have been so supportive of me during my years while battling cancer and writing this book I owe a deep debt of gratitude which cannot ever be fully paid and to my publisher, Mark McCullough of Wyndham Hall Press, who has always been my supporter and champion, I am eternally appreciative.

INTRODUCTION
A Specialization in Cancer Care and Treatment

This inquiry is of a psychiatric specialization which is not biomedical but rather psychosocial yet is a specialization practiced within the medical context of the care and treatment of cancer. Based on the principle that psychiatry is both a medical as well as a behavioral science, a point will be made of the interfacing of medical psychiatry and psychosocial psychiatry, the former in the tradition of Emil Kraepelin, M.D., (who contended that all mental illness was ultimately biochemical in nature) and the latter based on the work of Harry Stack Sullivan, M.D., called interpersonal psychotherapy (who demonstrated that most mental disorders are interpersonal in nature based on the hypothesis that "we are all simply more human than otherwise"). Since Freud established early on that psychoanalysis was a legitimate field of psychiatry within social psychology, the argument is dismissed here regarding whether or not psychiatry is exclusively biomedical or psychosocial in nature.

The intent here in these critical essays is, therefore, to offer a summary overview of the practice of the emotional care and treatment of cancer patients as a medical specialization within oncology which for reasons we will explain later we have labeled throughout as *psychiatric oncology*. Within this discussion, we will identify leading medical institutions and professional bodies in the United States which have chosen a range of labels for this specialization including *psycho-oncology, psychosocial oncology,* and *psych-oncology* as well as *psychiatric oncology*. We will explore the historic rise of this specialization during the past several decades and proceed to describe the various components of this specialization by plotting the psychosocial spectrum of cancer care within the general practice of oncology and the relationship of psychosocial and biomedical issues and challenges confronting this specialization.

Recognizing that there is both a scientific protocol in medical oncology as well as in psychiatric oncology, the inevitable issue of the interfacing of a scientific approach to the emotional care and treatment of the patient raises the issue of the spiritual character of the patient. The complex issues related to the faith-based care of the patient within a science-based institutional practice are broached within the context of the science of medicine and psychology. The enduring conundrum for the medical and behavioral sciences is how to engage with integrity and rationality in an enterprise in psychiatric oncology in which a majority of the practitioners (some studies suggest upwards of nearly 90%)–

doctors, nurses, administrators – embrace a firm belief in Divine Intervention within the context and framework of scientific practice and protocols. A discussion of the placebo effect of religious myth and metaphor in the face of the terminally ill involves patients as well as family and is considered herein.

(Note: I have not made an attempt to standardize the English usages in terms of spelling in this collection of essays owing to the range of sources from English-speaking scholars whose work from around the world has been utilized in this enquiry. I have chosen to honor each scholar's own English-language usage tradition even when within a single essay there are several variations.)

CHAPTER ONE

EMOTIONAL CARE AND TREATMENT OF THE CANCER PATIENT

The Oncology Specialization addressing the Psychosocial Dynamics of Healing

The emergence of this specialization in medical oncology addressing the emotional care of the patient, i.e., the psychological and social well-being of the individual diagnosed with cancer, has constituted a monumental advancement in the holistic care of the cancer patient. There has been a gradual but inevitable realization that the care of the total patient involves not only the biomedical side of a cancer diagnosis but the psychosocial side of the patient as well. This specialization indicates the recognition of the fundamental importance of the emotional matrix within the overall care of the cancer patient as well as family members and supporting medical staff within the health care community. Commencing early the 1970s at Memorial Sloan Kettering Cancer Center in New York under the leadership of Jimmie Holland, M.D., this Center sparked an accelerated development of the oncology community's realization that holistic care means not just biomedical but psychosocial well-being when dealing with a diagnosed patient with cancer (Holland, Bultz 2007) (See Appendix C).

During the last few years, the leading medical research hospitals and cancer centers across the U.S. have put in place an aggressive research and treatment agenda in the field of oncology designed to address specifically the behavioral components of cancer care (See Chapter Four). These institutions have come to recognize the central importance to the medical treatment of cancer of the emotional health issues confronting the patient undergoing a rapid behavioral matrix of shifts in feelings, attitudes, and emotional responsiveness to the diagnosis of cancer. The psychiatric community has particularly stepped up its involvement in the development of protocols incorporating the psychosocial aspects of oncology. One feature of this aggressive involvement is that of the nomenclature which inevitably has evolved when integrating complex psychiatric perspectives involved in oncological research and treatment. A lengthy discussion of the variances in labelling of this new specialization will include conflicting and contrasting characterizations of this specialization such as psycho-oncology, psychosocial oncology, psych-oncology, and most commonly psychiatric oncology (See Chapter Two for a lengthy discussion).

In the mid-late 1970s the oncology community was fully cognizant of the central importance of the emotional well-being of cancer patients and the recognition that depression and other behavioral stress-points play a central role in the overall trajectory of treatment and care through curative, palliative, and survival modalities of clinical oversight. Zabora and team (Zabora et al 2001) and Carlson and team (Carlson et al 2004) have shown through their clinical studies that there is most commonly an increase in emotional stress and depression at the commencement of a cancer diagnosis somewhat elevated above the normative population. Understandably, a predicable rise in anxiety-related behavioral distress results from the inevitable uncertainties which a diagnosis of cancer brings to the individual and the family involved not to mention the fears and stresses of what treatments are to be employed and the physical as well as emotional anxieties resulting from the unknown. Such factors as body-image and self-confidence in the face of changing physical demands and needs contribute to the prospects of a debilitating rush of depression. Fears of uncertainty as to the physical as well as emotional impact treatment modalities must be anticipated in the patient's overall sense of self and of well-being. Though the focus of much of psychiatric oncology research has been upon the impact depression and anxiety have upon the patient's response to the assessment, diagnosis, and treatment protocols, the Zabora and Carlson research team discovered to the surprise of many clinicians that some individuals are actually able to maintain a healthy balance of well-being during diagnosis and treatment and some studies even have reported an improvement in the overall sense of self and an improved self-image and social relationships on the part of the patient resulting from a cancer diagnosis.

In the early 1980s, research teams (Derogatis et al. 1983) were fully aware of the presence of depression and anxiety in the diagnosed patient and such findings contributed substantially to the increased interest within the medical community in the psychosocial character of cancer. Complementing the biomedical assessment and treatment of cancer was the increasing awareness of patient concerns regarding longevity, types and severity of treatments, and practical considerations regarding the anticipated increase in physical fatigue, emotional debilitation, physical characteristics such as nausea, hair loss, neuropathy and what was early on rather unfortunately labeled "chemo brain." In the past several decades, these concerns have been effectively integrated into the psychotherapeutic treatment of cancer patients and have become the core of psychiatric oncology. While Derogatis (1983) and colleagues have clinically verified that a majority of cancer patients do not actually experience a debilitating phase of depression and anxiety, the cancer diagnosis does produce a somewhat higher presence of these behavioral responses than within the normative population. Petticrew, Bell, and Hunter (2002) have found that the patient's anticipation of shorter survival rates and diminished psychological well-being are intimately connected and constitute a major focus of treatment within psychiatric oncology.

Early oncology care givers, physicians and nurses alike, were fully aware of the tremendously powerful impact a cancer diagnosis brings to the patient and, therefore, the range of emotional and behavioral responses to such a diagnosis constituted early on the primary focus of research by psycho-oncologists. Because of the complexity of physical and emotional features resulting from a cancer diagnosis, the patient is called upon to embrace a matrix of coping mechanisms to facilitate a mature response to the cancer diagnosis. Owing to the range of characteristics cancer brings to the patient, both physically and emotionally, there is the urgent need for the patient to have at his/her disposal coping mechanisms designed to mitigate the depression and anxiety which are inevitable. Roth and Cohen (1986) have identified early on a wide-reaching range of behavioral coping devices divided into two classifications, viz., approach-oriented coping and avoidance-oriented coping. Because they were among the earliest clinicians to identify and label these two classifications, there is the recognition that their researches have made a significant contribution to a deepening understanding of means of facilitating a healthy response to a cancer diagnosis on the part of the patient when assisted in the process of identification by the oncologists and treatment staff.

The early studies by Roth and Cohen (1986), in differentiating between approach coping, and avoidance coping have been extended through clinical studies over the past several decades and the findings have been helpful in assisting psychiatric oncologists and their colleagues in sorting out the variances in patient responses to diagnostic processes. *Approach coping*, explain the clinical data, assists the patient in identifying and embracing the cognitive, behavioral, and emotional factors involved in a diagnostic response which facilitates the patient's capacity to relate to the assessment and treatment modalities available to them while remaining engaged as a participant in the decision-making process shared with the care givers and the patient's family support unit. On the other hand, *avoidance coping* fosters a negativity regarding the assessment and diagnostic protocols thereby enforcing an emotional suppression of the reality of a cancer diagnosis resulting in a behavioral matrix which tends towards the elevation of social stress and anxiety. Navigating through this maze of confused feelings constitutes the grand challenge of psychiatric oncology.

Beyond "approach and avoidance" coping mechanisms, Stanton and team (2002) have labelled a behavioral response to a cancer diagnosis as "benefit finding" wherein the patient, upon learning of the presence of cancer, is called upon to identify within one's life those things which have up until the diagnosis been overlooked or undervalued. This "coping strategy," according to Stanton, provides a reflective opportunity for the patient to take stock of what really matters in life as against those daily frustrations which begin inevitably to recede in the face of a cancer diagnosis. Barskova (2009) has identified a point which he has labeled "post traumatic growth" wherein the individual, when confronted with the finality of a terminal diagnosis, is given an opportunity to readjust their relationship with friends and family and to assess what really matters in life on a daily basis. Another perspective is presented by Lee (2008) in which the individual, when confronting the demands of a life whose terminus is envisioned, provides an opportunity to pragmatically navigate that which is perceived to be truly existentially meaningful to the patient. Park and colleagues (2008) suggest in their clinical studies this "meaning making" endeavor can prove to constitute a real positive opportunity for emotional growth in the patient in the quest for a quality of life which has until the diagnosis been somewhat discounted or overlooked. In a subsequent essay dealing with the scope of interpersonal psychiatry, we will see how the major contributions of Harry Stack Sullivan serves very well this emphasis upon "meaning making" in which we explore the depth of significance in his statement: "We are all simply more human than otherwise." Also, it must be pointed out that the concept of the "will to meaning" constitutes the core of Viktor Frankl's logotherapeutic approach to human development as a counter-balance to Freud's "will to pleasure" and Adler's "will to power" (Morgan, 2017). The challenge is often, to especially a particularly productive individual who has been diagnosed with cancer, a fear of decline in self-worth owing to a diminishment of productivity along the lines of their life's trajectory of self-meaning. Often a drastic reassessment of the meaning of one's life is the result of the confrontation with a cancer diagnosis resulting in a decline in a level of productivity which has historically characterized the individual's own self-identity.

Though somewhat marginal to the primary focus of psychiatric oncology, concerns for behavioral responses to cancer diagnosis and treatment are buttressed by an overarching concern for pre-cancerous behaviors which are linked to cancer such as smoking and excess alcohol consumption as well as the popular attraction to cosmetic skin products which are themselves frequently dangerous. Psychiatric oncologists are fully cognizant of the negative behavioral choices made by individuals who do not have cancer but which may eventuate in a cancer diagnosis. According to Gotay (2005) attention to such behavioral choices falls within the spectrum of the psychiatric oncologist. The rightful concern for such behavior falls within the domain of psychiatric oncology owing to the inevitable need for behavior change when once a cancer has been diagnosed. Consedine and colleagues (2004) have emphasized the role of fear and anxiety in individuals failing to seek screening as a rational mechanism for cancer surveillance. Zeng and colleagues (2014) have called clinical attention specifically to the prevalence of physical fatigue (and cognitive exhaustion) as an exasperating characteristic of a cancer diagnosis and the call on the part of the attending physicians for diagnosed patients to assert themselves towards a meaningful and viable behavioral matrix. This orientation on the part of the patient can contribute to a deeper feeling of well-being in spite of fatigue and exhaustion.

The incremental development over the last several decades in the overall perception of what treatment means to cancer patients has to do with a shifting of focus from a passivity on the part of the patient to an active patient participatory engagement with the treatment team of nurses and oncologists. What was once thought of as merely patient compliance with the treatment team's assessment and treatment plan DiMatteo, Lepper, and Croghan (2000) have pointed out that the newly established protocol in the patient/doctor relationship is now calling for a more ethically oriented treatment plan involving collaboration rather than compliance between patient and doctor. This shift is now recognized as *adherence* rather than *compliance* and this has become increasingly the purview of psychiatric oncology. DiMatteo and colleagues (2000) have demonstrated in their clinical studies that the cognitive and behavioral causes of non-compliance on the part of the patient to the treatment protocol established by the medical team has to do with the absence of a sense of collaborative participation in the overall care of the cancer patient such that non-compliance commonly suggests a passive resistance to a treatment plan to which the patient has not been a planning participant.

In addition to misinformation or a lack of clarity on the part of the patient regarding the treatment plan, too often failure to comply to treatment adherence is the direct result of the patient's fear and/or experience of toxic side effects, lack of collaborative communication between the patient and the treatment team and protocol management, and behavioral and emotional factors resulting in depression and anxiety. In 2016, Greer and colleagues emphasized the presence of challenges confronting treatment adherence which has become a major focus of concern and research within the psychiatric oncology arena of cancer care owing to the increase utilization of oral antineoplastic drugs for patients who are taking chemotherapeutic medicines. These patients are often called upon to oversee the management of their own medical cocktails at home without nursing supervision. This elevated challenge placed upon the patient to self-monitor their oral medication has often, with measured success, replaced the traditional intravenous chemotherapeutic protocols administered in the chemotherapeutic theatre by the nursing staff.

Complementing the insights into the emotional and behavioral care of the cancer patients have been clinical researches conducted in the field called "health psychology" where there has been the elevated recognition that social support provided to the patient can lead to a strong psychological sense of well-being (Valtorta et al 2016). Recognizing that patients undergoing aggressive cancer treatment commonly benefit tremendously from social support networks such as family and friends, psychiatric oncologists have become increasingly pro-active in fostering social network support for patients particularly engaged in intrusive and complex treatment protocols which too often produce depression and anxiety in the absence of a strong social supportive network. It is universally recognized within oncological treatment protocols that there is frequently an emotional toll experienced by the patient undergoing intrusive and complex treatment modalities such that a strong social support network involving not only the medical team but the patient's own social network has shown in clinical studies to be most beneficial to the patient's responsiveness to the treatment plan. Nausheen and colleagues (2009) have shown in their clinical studies that such support both in instrumental and emotional matrices frequently result in an improved sense of self and well-being for the patient. Counter-balancing this emphasis upon the benefits of social network support is the clinical studies conducted by Lunstad and colleagues (2015) which have demonstrated that in cases where the cancer patient is confronted with an emotionally changed response to the diagnosis as a result of social isolation and loneliness, the self-image and sense of well-being on the part of the patient is greatly diminished such that a breakdown in family relations and the overall social network of support vanishes producing an elevation of a sense of "illness" rather than "health." Lundstad and colleagues have shown in their clinical studies that this encroachment of isolation and a diminishment of a sense of well-being results in a clinically documented negative impact upon the patient, both physically and emotionally.

Early on medical personnel involved in the treatment of cancer patients have been aware of the crucial importance of communication between the patient and that of the medical team of oncologists and nursing staff. The clinical documentation verifying the positive results of effective communication between these various social sub-sets – medical team and family – has been developed and clinically documented particularly well by Zolnierek and Dimatteo (2009). Various modalities of communication management structures, such as cognitive behavioral therapy, have proven most beneficial to the overall well-being and sense of self on the part of the cancer patient has also been documented in the Greer and team's clinical studies (2010). Waldron and team (2013) have shown clinical evidence that the quality of life is enhanced by effective communication between patient and care givers positively affecting both the patient and the medical team. Gabriel and team (2020) have further demonstrated through clinical studies that the well-being of the "entire family" is greatly facilitated through effective patient/medical team communication.

The broad field of health psychology has significantly contributed not only to a deepening understanding of the relevance of psychosocial factors affecting cardiovascular disease but increasingly the application of these insights into the psychosocial care and treatment of cancer patients as well. Hanahan and Weinberg (2011) have shown in their studies a direct correlation between biological processes and psychological factors integrated in the overall care of the cancer patient. The interactive relationship between bio-behavioral pathways and treatment modalities on the part of the cancer patient greatly enhances the prospects of a positive psychological outcome to the patient's sense of well-being during treatment (Antoni et al 2006). Bower and Lamkin (2013) have clinically demonstrated that such factors as pain and fatigue are substantially mitigated by a bio-behavioral sensitivity to treatment which involves the patient's social network.

Thanks to the careful clinical studies of leading psychiatric oncologists and psychotherapists in the field of behavioral mood studies related to both depression and anxiety disorders, there is growing awareness that the acceleration of emotional stressors can be directly linked to a diagnosis of cancer in a patient. Many misperceptions and "common maladaptive cognitions" linked to a cancer diagnosis include a misunderstanding of the nature of contingent pain and related physical discomforts as the patient experiences the inevitable progression of the carcinoma. Of particular concern are the resulting anxieties which emerge following a diagnosis and the commencement of treatment of cancer which directly impact the patient's sense of well-being and quality of life (Osborn, Demoncada, Feueerstein, 2006). Osborn and colleagues have clinically demonstrated that cognitive behavioral therapy and related psychotherapies have proven to be especially effective in the management of the patient's anxieties and depression. As used by trained psychiatric oncologists, these various psychotherapies have shown that their use in the management of chronic pain and physical as well as emotional fatigue which commonly results from the use of chemotherapy and radiation can prove particularly effective in assisting the patient to more significantly manage their own well-being and their sense of self in the face of otherwise debilitating pain and depression (Syrjala et al 2014; Kwekkeoom et al 2010).

The Sloan Kettering Cancer Center research team under the leadership of Dr. Jimmie Holland early on realized that social prejudices which characterize psychological oversight and intervention in the care of cancer patients tended to produce a substantial impediment to clinical studies which psychiatric oncologists developed in the 1970s and 1980s in spite of the professional prejudices present at the time. As recent as 2018, the National Comprehensive Cancer Studies continued aggressively to push for regular screening of cancer patients through a protocol of diagnosis, treatment, and survivorship. These studies, it was shown, demonstrated conclusively that patients suffering from depression and anxiety benefited emotionally from psychosocial assessments of the patient's life prospects, sense of well-being, and overall adjustments to the inevitabilities of a cancer diagnosis including living with cancer, cancer-free survivorship issues, and the transition to the end of life care. Thanks to the emergence of psychiatric oncology growing out of the numerous cancer research centers around the country, the prejudice and stigma attached to the diagnostic, assessment, and treatment protocols have been essentially dispelled in professional practice with such success as to stifle any significant on-going criticism of this work in the field of psychiatric oncology.

CHAPTER TWO
THE LABELING OF PSYCHIATRIC ONCOLOGY

Its Meaning and History

In science, the labeling of things is crucially important for precision and for universal standardization and particularly within the practice of medicine and psychiatry. The history of science is the history of labeling and the evolution of scientific precision is reflected in this process. When Eugene Bleuler changed the name of Arnold Pick's "dementia praecox" to "schizophrenia" in 1911, he set the stage for Emil Kraepelin who popularized the new more descriptive term to the advantage of practicing psychiatrists. The labeling process, however, is fraught with pitfalls and missteps as well. It is agreed within the field of psychotherapy that Freud's development of the term "psychoanalysis" constitutes the quintessentially exact description of what his clinical practice involved. Alfred Adler, however, was left with something less than descriptively helpful with the term "Individual Psychology" while Carl Jung had nothing more than "Analytical Psychology." Both of these schools of thought were always perceived, and to their chagrin, as mere variants of psychoanalysis *per se.* The developmental emergence of psychotherapy schools of thought reflected in the labels which sought to describe what were the variant nuances of analysis is reflected in such a wide array of labels today as transactional analysis, cognitive behavior therapy, client-centered therapy, etc., etc., etc. To-date, the American Psychological Association records upwards of 400 different labels for variant modalities of treatment within the broad field of psychotherapy (Morgan, 2020: 237).

The history of the labeling of psychiatry is not our concern here but that the term has undergone over the last century and a half a transmogrification is indisputable (Shorter, 1997; Allexander and Selesnick, 1977; Browne and Burton, 2016). It is generally agreed, however, that Emil Kraepelin's development of a biological or organic description of psychiatric practice constitutes the first formalized biomedical model based on an emerging molecular biology and the eventuality of psychopharmacology. This form of psychiatry was predicated on the conviction that mental disorders were essentially biological. The emergence of psychosocial psychiatry emerged with the coming of the social sciences, interpersonal theories of personality, and psychoanalysis such that mental disorders were classified in terms of a behavioral matrix rather than a biological one (Morgan, 2015; 2021). Whereas psychopharmacology grew out of a biological focus in medical psychiatry, psychotherapy developed from a cognitive focus leading to a duality of psychiatric practice, i.e., both medical and psychosocial. In psychopharmacology, the treatment focused upon behavioral modifications leading to practical functionality of the patient whereas in the psychotherapeutic form of psychiatry the focus centered squarely upon the causality of mental disorders which produces dysfunctional behavior.

A classic sub-set within psychiatry in which the challenge of labeling is evident is that of the non-medical treatment of cancer. The emergence of what in the last few decades has come to be called variously psychiatric oncology, psychosocial oncology, and psycho-oncology is illustrative of the labeling challenge. Oncology is the care and treatment of patients with cancer and there is a full recognition, based on years of clinical study, that the biomedical treatment of the cancer patient is greatly enhanced if the emotional and social well-being of the patient is taken full cognizance of in the overall treatment plan. The tempest in the tea pot (and on occasion an internecine battle) over which is the more appropriate label for this emotional and social focus in oncological care and treatment of the patient centers around whether or not and to what extent the use of the label "psychiatric" is correctly indicative of this mode of care and treatment. It has been cogently argued that "psycho-oncology" is the least desirable label given the popular misuse of the term "psycho" when applied to a variety of behaviors in the lay media. Psychosocial oncology is correctly suggestive of the focus on the emotional and interpersonal dynamic in cancer care and treatment and the argument for this label is strong. However and finally, since the practice of this aspect of cancer care occurs within the arena of a medical environment such as a hospital or a cancer clinic, and given the recognition that the label "psychiatry" implies a professional level of competency paralleling the medical oncologist, there is a reigning argument that "psychiatric oncology" should be the standard of reference. When full recognition that psychiatry focuses upon both the biomedical as well as the emotional and behavioral well-being of the patient, the case is generally recognized as sufficient to justify the label "psychiatric oncology." A precedent set for the use of the term psychiatry in describing a range of behavioral protocols in the field of medical care was earlier established with the development of the formalized professional body, namely, that of psychiatric nursing, which incorporated the psychosocial aspects of care and treatment within the context of the medical care of cancer patients. It is not inconsequential here to call attention to the fact that Dr. Jimmie C. Holland of the Sloan Kettering

Cancer Center held during her faculty tenure a professorship titled the Wayne E. Chapman Chair in Psychiatric Oncology (See Appendix C).

Given the cultural importance within the *zeitgeist* of "getting the job done" in modern society, the heavy emphasis has shifted from an earlier psychotherapeutically informed desire for treatment of the cause of mental disorders to a biomedical treatment of the behavioral complex producing dysfunction. Whereas the psychosocial form of psychiatry relies heavily upon the psychotherapeutic treatment requiring time and financial investment in clinical counseling, the biomedical form of psychiatry relies upon the psychopharmacological interventions developed to modify behavior while sidestepping the emotional causes of dysfunction. The advantage of this approach to the treatment of mental disorders is a minimum of time investment on the part of the patient and psychiatrist and the ready availability of short-term effective pharmaceuticals developed by the industry for the "quick fix." Psychotherapeutic psychiatry is expensive in time and money whereas medical psychiatry is inexpensive requiring a minimum of time on the part of both patient and psychiatrist and a minimal medical cost for psychotropic medication. The ideal treatment plan is an integrative approach using both psychotherapy and pharmaceuticals under oversight by a team of psychosocial psychiatry and biomedical psychiatry. To reach an understanding that these two perspectives are not intrinsically competitive but complementary is the fundamental responsibility of the medical team. The impediment to this holistic approach is a monumental expense to the patient, the medical team, and the host institution. In a word, psychotherapy is costly; pharmaceuticals are much less so.

It is not our intention in the following chapters to imply that the practice of psychiatric oncology requires the practitioner to be both a psychologist and an oncologist. However, the following extended discussion of Emil Kraepelin's descriptive psychiatry and Harry Stack Sullivan's interpersonal psychiatry is presented here to both emphasize and delineate the efficacy of the oncology team's general knowledge of the relationship between the biomedical character of cancer as well as the psychosocial spectrum of cancer patient care. It is hoped that a brief overview of the relationship between and an understanding of descriptive psychiatry and personality developmental theory might prove beneficial to the treatment team in their care of the cancer patient – not just the carcinoma but the actual personal as well.

CHAPTER THREE
THE SCOPE OF DESCRIPTIVE PSYCHIATRY
(Emil Kraepelin, M.D., in profile)

As we have been pointing out throughout this inquiry, psychiatric oncology is based upon the two-fold convergence of the biogenic and psychogenic understanding of the nature of psychiatry as a medical specialization. Without an understanding of the binary function of psychiatry, there can be no real grasp of the central importance and fundamental function of psychiatric oncology. Though a history of psychiatry and its relationship to both psychotherapy and psychopharmacology has been done elsewhere (Morgan, 2021), it is fundamentally important to understand here the historical interfacing of biogenic psychiatry as developed by Emil Kraepelin, M.D., and the rise to central importance of psychogenic psychiatry as developed by Harry Stack Sullivan, M.D. Out of this fruitful relationship has evolved the medical and social science foundations for psychiatric oncology. I have taken this time in the following chapters to elaborate upon the fundamentals of biogenic psychiatry as developed by Kraepelin and psychogenic psychiatry as developed by Sullivan owing to the void in general knowledge of these two branches of modern psychiatry and their relevance to the birth and growth of psychiatric oncology which grew out of the work initially introduced by Jimmie Holland, M.D., at the Sloan Kettering Cancer Center (Appendix C).

Any creditable study of contemporary psychiatry and its relationship to psychopathology and psychopharmacology, to say nothing of psychotherapy, must begin with a consideration of the profound influence Emil Kraepelin has had upon both the development of biological psychiatry and its relevance to the discussion of the relationship between medicine and psychotherapy (Morgan, 2021). Certainly the recognized founder (or the primary one) of modern biogenic psychiatry as well as psychopharmacology, i.e., Emil Kraepelin, M.D., must be credited with having brought together biology and psychology within the framework of a biogenic psychiatry such that the history of the disciplines of psychiatry and psychopharmacology cannot be written without an understanding of his early and dominating prominence.

As the founder of modern biogenic psychiatry as well as psychopharmacology, Emil Kraepelin (1856-1926) was a German psychiatrist driven by the conviction that the fundamental nature of psychiatric illness and disease is biologically and genetically linked as an organic dysfunction. Dismissing demonic superstition, Kraepelin, as a dedicated clinician and medical researcher, was convinced as to the genetic and biological origins of most mental disorders labeled and treated as "mental disease" rather than as merely psychogenic disorders. His perspective and clinical orientation has reigned supreme from the beginning of the 20th century in Europe as well as in America. In spite of the psychodynamic innovations brought about by the development of Sigmund Freud's psychoanalysis, organic psychiatry has at the beginning of the 21st century found a resurgence of interest within the psychiatric community substantially due to the rise and influence of the pharmaceutical industry and the development of psychotropic medications which reflect the influence of Kraepelin. Shortened treatment time and reduced treatment costs in medication constitute the two driving forces in modern psychiatric treatment.

The search for a systemic classification scheme in the practice of psychiatry constituted the driving force in the life's work of Kraepelin. Though he has been justifiably criticized for an eclectic style of gathering data for his studies, often from non-medically linked sources, his commitment to a method whereby mental disease, as he described it and understood it, constitutes one of the great contributions to the advancement of mental health studies in modern times. The scope of his quest was expansive and the intent was to create a comprehensive taxonomic classification system to serve the needs of the psychiatric community. Even today, his efforts are celebrated as epic.

Coming from relatively humble circumstances in which his father, Karl Wilhelm Kraepelin, was an opera singer turned music teacher, Emil Kraepelin was born in the German town of Neustrelitz in 1856, three years before Darwin published his *On the Origin of Species.* Thanks to his older brother, Karl, Emil was made acquainted with the science of biology which occupied his interest and attention for the remainder of his life. His brother Karl was destined to become the Director of the Hamburg Zoological Museum and Emil was on his way to revolutionizing modern psychiatry. Beginning at the University of Leipzig in 1874 and concluding his medical studies in 1878 at the University of Wurzburg, Kraepelin was privileged to have studied with the leading scientists of the day at Leipzig, including Paul Fleschsig in neuropathology, and experimental psychology with Wilhelm Wundt, under whom Kraepelin produced a major research paper titled "The Influence of Acute Illness in the Causation of Mental Disorders," which launched his career in psychiatry. Completing his training and examinations for his medical degree in 1878, authorizing him to practice medicine, he went on to the University of Munich where he worked under Bernhard von Gudden from

1878 to 1882. He completed his doctorate at the University of Leipzig in 1883 while working in Wundt's psychopharmacology laboratory with a doctoral dissertation titled "The Place of Psychology in Psychiatry."

The major publication of his career argued that psychiatry was a branch of medical science. Sigmund Freud, on the other hand, later argued that psychiatry is a sub-set of psychology, not medicine (Morgan, 2021). Kraepelin's book which went through several editions is credited with having established him as the leader in the field of developing psychiatry. Published in 1883, it was initially titled *Compendium of Psychiatry: For the Use of Students and Physicians (Psychiatrie: Zum Gebrauche fur Stradirende und Aertze),* appearing subsequently in multiple volumes under the title *A Textbook: Foundations of Psychiatry and Neuroscience* (*Ein Lehrbuch der Psychiatrie*). Psychiatry's rightful place within the medical sciences was based on his insistence that its mission is to observe and experiment in the natural sciences, addressing issues related to the physical causes of mental illness, with the intent of establishing a taxonomy of mental disease. The monumental goal and aspiration of this new trajectory of psychiatry as envisioned by Kraepelin was the plotting of case histories of mental disorders to reach the ability to predict the development of various types of mental illnesses, factoring in personal data of the patient.

In recognition of the creative energies expended in proposing this accelerated development of a modern psychiatry based on case studies, Kraepelin in 1884 became the top medical professional in the Prussian town of Leubus followed the next year by being made Director of Dresden's Treatment and Nursing Institute. In 1886 at age 30, Kraepelin became Professor of Psychiatry at the University of Dorpat in Estonia where, as director of the 80-bed University Clinic, he launched his monumental data-base study of clinical case histories attempting to track the development of mental illnesses in his patients based on his emerging classification system of mental disease. Four years later he was named to the Chairmanship of the Department of Psychiatry at the University of Heidelberg where he stayed until 1903 when he became Professor of Clinical Psychiatry in the University of Munich. Within five years he was elected to membership in the Royal Swedish Academy of Sciences, and in 1912 established a research center which eventually became in 1917 the German Institute for Psychiatric Research. Seven years later it was incorporated into the Kaiser Wilhelm Society for the Advancement of Science including its own Kraepelin-designed research building funded in 1928 by the

Rockefeller Foundation. This initiative was at the request of the German Association for Psychiatry of which he was head from 1906-1920 combined with funding from a Jewish German-American named James Loeb.

Kraepelin took advantage of his international reputation to challenge the current practices of psychiatric institutions at the time in their treatment of mentally ill patients particularly protesting against psychiatric asylums and the tendency to imprison as criminals rather than medically treat as patients those suffering from mental illness. A point which will prove relevant as we pursue the treatment options employed in psychiatric oncology later in this book, Kraepelin was outspoken in his criticism of psychotherapeutic theories which were based, as in Freudian psychoanalysis, on the notion of early sexuality as the cause of mental illness. Kraepelin rather preferred, in his rejection of philosophical speculations, to concentrate his research attention upon clinical case histories, and not inconsequentially, the significance of neuropathology in the development of his taxonomic scheme.

Emphasizing the distinction between his own approach to the study of mental illness which he called "clinical," in contrast to the popular method at the time which he labelled "symptomatic," this paradigm shift set the stage for the development of his taxonomic scale which included hundreds of what he chose to characterize as mental diseases. He employed a new term in this classification system which he called "syndrome" defined as common patterns of symptoms over time thereby elevating the sophistication of psychiatric practice. He was convinced, based on his own clinical studies, that he had made a monumental advance in the field of psychiatry by having moved away from the common practice of symptomatic classification of mental illness to that of a clinical perspective based rather upon taxonomic classifications which take into account the conditions of the origin, progress, and termination of each clinical case of mental illness.

Indicative of the creative brilliance of Kraepelin's quest for a taxonomic solution to the diagnostic challenges in psychiatry at the time was the development of what has become known as the Kraepelinian dichotomy. In this development, he proposed two types of psychosis rather than a unitary type, i.e., *manic depression* (now covering recurrent major depression as well as bipolar disorder) and *dementia praecox* (now known as schizophrenia thanks to the popularizing of it by Dr. Eugen Bleuler, Freud's colleague). The creation of the descriptive term of *dementia praecox* grew out of his insistence that the criteria for the labeling of a mental illness is that of a predictability of outcome and prognosis describing a peculiar condition of what he called a mental weakness which emerges in childhood. Eventually by 1899 the term had been so well received within common clinical practice as sufficiently descriptive as to incorporate *catatonia*, *dementia paranoides*, as well as *hebephrenia*. A fundamentally operational methodology developed by Kraepelin was based on the recognition that any particular symptom may at any time be evidenced in any one of these three disorders. Therefore, it behooved him to point out that the distinction of each separate disease in terms of symptoms rather than the causal pathology is not based on a pathognomonic symptom but rather upon a pattern of symptoms. At the time there existed no physiological or genetic text for verification of a diagnosis. The Kraepelin style of diagnostics, then, is based upon an identifiable pattern of symptoms rather than the old style of identifying a mental disorder based on the grouping of complimenting symptoms.

Illustrations of this demonstrable verification of pattern identity were found in the genetic composition of these mental disorders seen in the course and outcome of the recognized pattern. So, for instance, there is clinical evidence that schizophrenia more commonly appears within the familial matrix of relatives of an individual diagnosed with schizophrenia than otherwise. The same is true of manic depression as well as bipolar disorders. Though today researchers are not willing to go so far as to contend for the genetic propensity of repetition, it must be pointed out that there is always the possibility that socio-environmental factors may contribute to this phenomenon of frequency. Believing that schizophrenia reflects a patterned tracking of etiology, Kraepelin demonstrated with clinical evidence a propensity to developmental deterioration of the mental capacity of the patient manifested as either a graded or erratic decline. However, in the case of manic depression, the patient experiences intermittent decline with episodic periods of no evident symptoms of the disorder. The incremental, often erratic, and predictably episodic manifestation of symptoms led Eugen Bleuler, Freud's colleague, in an effort to correct Kraepelin, to rename *dementia praecox* "schizophrenia," thereby indicating the clinically verified fact that mental decline among such patients was not inevitable, whereas the "dementia" term had suggested the irreversible nature of such mental decline.

By 1920, Kraepelin had fully accepted the corrective and went so far as to suggest that in recognition of the diagnostic connectivity of manic depression and schizophrenia that there should be a new category of designation labelled "schizoaffective disorder." The etiology of both *dementia praecox* and *manic depression* was a major concern of Kraepelin though he wrote little about his researches involving these two mental illnesses. Yet, from 1896 until his death 30 years later, he continued to believe that schizophrenia in particular would be clinically proven to result from a systemic metabolic disease process impacting the human anatomy, particularly the brain, in a cataclysmic onslaught of terminal symptoms.

Kraepelin's development as a research scientist and clinician can be followed through the various editions of his major textbook, *Compendium of Psychiatry* (1883), with which he both launched his career and continued to accelerate his achievements. His book became the textbook for psychiatry at the time constituting the primary resource for diagnostic classification of mental illness, but other forms of disorders beyond schizoaffective disorders appeared, such as in his 6th edition as a category called "moral insanity." A personality disorder affecting the moral sensibilities of the patient without the presence of either delusions or hallucinations led Kraepelin to define this classification as the absence of sensibilities which normally serve to counter-balance the unacceptable demands of egoism labelled "degenerative" by Kraepelin. The old term devised by Cesare Lombroso was called "born criminal," but Kraepelin reconfigured the diagnostic description to reflect a moral defect without the necessity of identifying any distinguishing physical characteristics.

The movement in Kraepelin's textbook from "moral insanity" to "born criminal" occurred in 1904 reallocating it from the classification of "congenital feeble-mindedness" to a completely new category labeled "Psychopathic personalities," characterized by a degenerative theory of devolution. Liking this new arrangement and suggestive of his taxonomic classifications, he proposed four different types, namely, born criminals thought of as "inborn delinquents," pathological liars, querulous persons, and *Triebmenschen* (compulsive behavior of vagabonds, spendthrifts, and dipsomaniacs). Though Kraepelin did not have clinical evidence suggesting an actual congenital cause, leaving his assessment to be strictly biogenic, it was the German psychiatrist Julius Ludwig August Koch who proposed the classification term "psychopathic inferiorities" suggesting that both congenital and acquired types could be identified diagnostically. In light of the problematic impression that Kraepelin was suggesting a moral sense being inborn and static, his position has been discounted by today's psychiatric community as essentially promoting a notion of a moral defect instead of a positive drive towards criminal behavior. The criticism of his nosology was of it being a reductionistic roster of an unacceptable behavioral matrix instead of a *bona fide* medical condition. However, many diagnostic components still continue in the *Diagnostic and Statistical Manual (DSM)* and *The International Classification of Diseases and Related Health Problems (ICD-10* as reference sources related to the psychopathology of personality disorders.

Early in the development of his classic textbook in psychiatry, Kraepelin had employed the term "psychopathic" rather generously from 1896 within which he included compulsive insanity, impulsive insanity, homosexuality, and mood disturbances of a variety of kinds and sorts. However, in less than a decade he had chosen to sophisticate his labeling by employing a more diagnostically descriptive characterization of mental disturbances including suggesting that the presenting disease characteristics could more descriptively be categorized as "psychopathic personalities." By the 8th edition of his textbook in 1909 Kraepelin had elevated this suggestion to a separate roster of behavioral matrices including a distinctive "dissocial" type of psychopathic personality, such as what he labeled "the unstable," the *Triebmenschen* motivated individual, eccentrics, the liars and swindler, and the perennially quarrelsome. Clearly before his time, Kraepelin actually assessed mood disturbances as merely an extension of manic depression which is most common today.

Believing that underlying each of the more conspicuous psychiatric disorders, Kraepelin suggested that a biological or brain pathology constituted the fundamental foundations of such. With his colleague Alois Alzheimer, he was a co-discoverer of the Alzheimer's disease, his university laboratory actually making the discovery of the pathology leading to that disease. However, following his 1903 move to the University of Munich as Professor of Clinical Psychiatry, he turned increasingly to issues related to social policy and their relationship to medical science research.

Without doubt, Kraelepin's monumental contribution to modern psychiatry cannot be discounted and his taxonomic system of classification of mental illness has stood the test of time, albeit periodically revised based on increasingly sophisticated clinical data. Though his pioneering work in schizophrenia and manic depression is seldom referenced today, the 20th century often saw the unjustified dismissal of his organic psychiatric model owing to the onslaught of Freudian psychoanalytic theory and the rise of the professional non-medical psychotherapeutic community, particularly in the United States. However, his basic theories regarding the diagnostic classification and treatment of psychiatric disorders are evidenced, often without credit, in the major reference and resource textbooks created by the American Psychiatric Association in the *Diagnostic and Statistical Manual of Mental Disorders (5th Edition)* and the World Health Organization in the *International Classification of Diseases* system.

The transition from a biogenic psychiatry to a psychogenic psychiatry occurred in the early-mid 19th century thanks greatly to the rise of psychodynamic psychotherapy and particularly Freudian psychoanalysis (Morgan, 2020). This shift from biomedical to psychosocial emphasis within psychiatric practice would eventually swing back owing to the rise of psychopharmacology. However, the impact the psychosocial emphasis had thanks to Freud, Jung, Adler, and Maslow would leave a lasting mark upon psychiatric practice. This reality would be most profoundly evidenced in the life's work of the psychiatrist, Harry Stack Sullivan, M.D.

CHAPTER FOUR
THE SCOPE OF INTERPERSONAL PSYCHIATRY
(Harry Stack Sullivan, M.D., in profile)

Since the mid-1900s, a leading school of theory and practice within psychotherapy has been a variation on psychoanalytic or psychodynamic psychotherapy called "interpersonal or social psychiatry" developed by Harry Stack Sullivan, M.D. At the young age of sixteen, he attended Cornell University to which he had won a scholarship from the State of New York and then proceeded to the Chicago College of Medicine and Surgery from which he grated in 1917.

Subsequent to graduation with his medical degree and in an effort to establish himself, he worked with schizophrenic patients at various hospitals, demonstrating a notable capacity to bring some success in dealing with schizophrenics using what he was already calling "interpersonal therapy." This interpersonal therapeutic approach he was developing involved the training of staff to enact safe, corrective interpersonal interactions with the patients, contending as he did that the normative institutional hospital environment was artificial and counterproductive to personality development. He subsequently served as a staff physician in the U.S. Army but two years later, he landed a position at the St. Elizabeths Hospital in Washington, D.C, the first federally funded psychiatric hospital in the U.S. Without any previous training in psychiatry whatsoever, Sullivan was most fortunate in working with the notable Dr. William Alanson White, an early and successful psychiatrist trained in the Freudian school of psychoanalysis. Additionally, clinical research at Sheppard and Enoch Pratt Hospital consumed a portion of Sullivan's life and passion from 1923 to 1930 as did a brief appointment in the University of Maryland's School of Medicine. He quickly established a reputation for successfully treating patients diagnosed with schizophrenia and began to write and publish his research findings based on his clinical studies (Freedheim, 1992).

During what Sullivan called his "Baltimore period" of theoretical development, he was engaged in extensive clinical experience and reach with institutionalized schizophrenics. It was here that he began to think about interpersonal relations as a key ingredient in the therapeutic treatment of the mentally ill. In attempting to decipher the nonsensical speech of the schizophrenic, he realized that their illness was a means of coping with anxiety generated from a social or interpersonal environment rather than of biogenic origins (Zeig, 1987).

By 1931, Sullivan was sufficiently well-known and

established to be asked to participate, indeed, even head up an initiative which led to the creation of the Washington School of Psychiatry. At this time he moved to New York where he developed a large and lucrative private practice and, interestingly enough, underwent 300 hours of psychoanalysis himself from Dr. Clara Thompson, a well-established Freudian therapist. In later years, he was both a professor and head of the department of psychiatry at the Georgetown University Medical School and subsequently served as the president of the William Alanson White Psychiatric Foundation. Part of his role was to serve as editor of a newly created and soon to be considered internationally distinguished journal, *Psychiatry*, commenced in 1938, while simultaneously serving as chairman of the council of Fellows of the Washington School of Psychiatry. During these very productive years, he became a colleague and friend of Edward Sapir, a cultural anthropologist, and Harold Lasswell, a political scientist, both from the University of Chicago. Of special relevance to his theory-building enterprise of international relations was his friendship with George Herbert Mead, Robert Ezra Park, and W. I. Thomas, all international distinguished sociologists at the University of Chicago (Morgan, 2017). Other major figures with whom he came in contact and with whom he established personal friendships included such professionally distinguished persons as Karen Horney, Erich Fromm, Frieda Fromm-Reichmann, and of special mention is Adolf Meyer. These experiences greatly broadened Sullivan's grasp of the behavioral and social sciences which eventually had a profound effect upon his theory of personality. In 1949, at age 57, he died of a persistent cardiovascular disease.

Ten years before Sullivan's death, the William Alanson White Foundation decided that a series of lectures should be given to honor the memory of White, a colleague of Sullivan's, who had died in 1937, and, of course, Sullivan was chosen to give the first series (Sullivan, 1953). He actually gave five lectures to small groups in an auditorium in a building owned by the Department of the Interior in Washington, DC. In these lectures, Sullivan made his first public attempt to present both a comprehensive and well-thought-out explanation of his concept of personality development including psychiatric disorders and treatment. In February of 1940, they were all published in the journal, *Psychiatry*, at the insistence of Sullivan's friends and colleagues, but against his best judgment. He was not pleased with his performance but finally consented and they appeared. Not surprisingly, they attracted much attention within the psychiatric and social science communities and in the following years many mental health and social science professional workers wrote to secure copies of this issue of the periodical.

"Psychiatry," Sullivan had written, "is the study of processes that involve or go on between people. The field of psychiatry is the field of interpersonal relations, under any and all circumstances in which these relations exist" (Sullivan, 1953). This is the thesis set forth by Sullivan in his work, where he expressed the central ideas of his theory of personality. Through his development of the theory, he made not only a vital contribution in the treatment of mental disorder -- in particular, schizophrenia -- but he opened an entirely new approach to the study of human personality (Mullahy, 1970). In the view of many analysts, he made the most original contribution to psychiatry since Freud. Rollo May has gone on record as saying, "As Freud was the prophet for the Victorian age of sexual suppression, Sullivan is the prophet for our schizoid age -- our age of unrelatedness, in which, beneath all the chatter of radio and newspapers and all the multitudes of 'contact,' people are often strangers to each other." Sullivan's book, *Conceptions of Modern Psychiatry* consists of reprints of the first William Alanson White Memorial Lectures, delivered by Sullivan in 1939, as has already been mentioned. They are profound and open a whole new world of interpretation of the nature of personality and as a science of interpersonal relations.

In this major work, Sullivan created a new viewpoint which is known today as the "interpersonal theory of psychiatry" (Freedheim, 1992). Sullivan's fundamental emphasis related to a theory of personality which is a "relatively enduring pattern of recurrent interpersonal situations which characterize a human life." Radically shifting from the psychoanalytic focus on the unconscious, Sullivan brought to his clinical research and practice a behavioral and social science perspective which had not been considered a significant component of personality theory until he did it himself. He argued that the concept of "personality" is itself a hypothetical entity which cannot be isolated from interpersonal situations and, indeed, interpersonal behavior is all that is observable about personality (Morgan, 2018). The rest, he suggests, is strictly metaphorical speculation and creative imagery. It is futile and fruitless to speak of a person's personality outside the social interactive matrix of the living person. Not discounting the significance of heredity and the maturation process affected by the physical environment, the real thing that determines the nature of a human person is social interaction with others (Sullivan, 1964). Of this, Sullivan was very insistent and unrelenting.

Never before had such an attempt been made to merge psychiatry and social psychology. Psychiatric oncology constitutes the most profound example of the development within psychiatry in the past forty years and the relevance of Sullivan's insights into interpersonal psychiatry cannot be over-emphasized. His theory of personality is the product of such a merger and it is greatly enriched by his acquaintance with and utilization of the social sciences. He writes: "The general science of psychiatry seems to me to cover much the same field as that which is studied by social psychology, because scientific psychiatry has to be defined as the study of interpersonal relations, and this in the end calls for the use of the kind of conceptual framework that we now call *field theory*. From such a standpoint, personality is taken to be hypothetical. That which can be studied is the pattern of processes which characterize the interaction of personalities in particular recurrent situations or fields which include the observer" (Sullivan, 1956). This attitude about the place and relevance of the "observer" in the clinical situation became a benchmark of Sullivan's innovative approach to the therapeutic encounter. He was, of course, influenced by the science philosopher, Heisenberg, on this point particularly in which Heisenberg developed in his concept of the "uncertainty principle."

Modern psychiatry as defined and practiced by Sullivan consisted of a study of personality characteristics which can be directly observed in the context of interpersonal relationships (Livesley and Larson, 2018). Systems of psychiatry based on statements about what is going on in the patient's mind are therefore similar to a system of thought which is built on axioms such as "All events are controlled by Divine Providence." The truth or falseness of this statement cannot be established by things that reasonably well educated people can see, hear, and feel. Much human experience can be cited to support such a statement, and much human experience can be cited to nullify it, but it is so set up that it must always remain a matter of faith. For Sullivan, a "personality characteristic" is defined as a thing which people can see, hear, and feel in their relationships with other individuals. This is the most fundamental working hypothesis in his personality theory (Sullivan, 1965). We have learned in psychiatric oncology that the understanding of the moods of the patient, the often impending depression and frequently anxiety, can best be addressed when the attending medical staff have a knowledge of the fundamentals of personality theory and the functional efficacy of interpersonal relations theory. A conjoining of the biogenic with the psychogenic character of mental health constitutes the most important foundation upon which to build an emotionally responsive acceptance of a cancer diagnosis on the part of the patient.

Though Sullivan is only willing to allow personality

to be purely hypothetical apart from the actually observable reality of social interaction, he does assert that it is a dynamic center of various processes which occurs in a series of interpersonal fields. This "dynamism" is a key concept in his overall personality theory. He give significant place to these processes by identifying and naming them as he constructs a platform of their characteristics. These processes, then, are *dynamisms*, *personifications*, the *self-system*, and *cognitive processes*. Let's explore each briefly here as they constitute the backbone of his major work, *Conceptions of Modern Psychiatry*, and facilitates an understanding of the relevance of Sullivan and interpersonal theory to psychiatric oncology.

The smallest unit of study in interpersonal relationships is what Sullivan calls "dynamism." It constituted an energy transference which meant any unit of behavior, either an actual act or a mental experience. These behavioral units become habitual ways of acting which involve the physical body of the person, such as the mouth, hands, arms, legs, etc. These dynamisms can then be broken down into a plethora of subsets, such as the fear, intimacy, etc. The dynamisms which are distinctively human in character are those which characterize one's interpersonal relations and function primarily to satisfy some basic needs of the individual. Three major dynamisms, according to

Sullivan, are malevolence, lust, and intimacy. Malevolence is the driving dynamism that one is living among one's own personal enemies and, if this negative dynamism emerges early in a child's life, he may find it difficult ever in adulthood to reach a fully trusting relationship with another person. Sullivan expressed it poignantly: "Once upon a time everything was lovely, but that was before I had to deal with people." Lust is another driving dynamism of the individual. Lust for Sullivan consists of the complex urges, feelings, and interpersonal actions which involve genital sexual activity as their distant or immediate goal. Lust begins in early adolescence.

Sullivan rejected the Freudian concept of sexuality and suggested that it was more or less inconsequential in childhood and early adolescence, but lust constitutes a major driving force in later adolescence. Intimacy for Sullivan is potentially a profoundly positive dynamism (Morgan, 2021). It occurs when the well-being of another person is as important to an individual as his own well-being. Intimacy does not occur in parent-child relationships and does not involve lust or sexual behavior and, Sullivan explains, it occurs only between members of the same sex. Lust becomes, then, a contaminant of intimacy for lust seeks to serve itself rather than the other person.

Personifications consist of an image that an

individual has of himself or of some other person. It is a complex of feelings, attitudes, and conceptions that grows out of experience with need-satisfaction and anxiety. Sullivan speaks often of the "good-mother," "bad-mother," and "overprotective mother" as examples. When these personifications are shared by a large social grouping, they become stereotypes such as "all Irishman are drunks," "all Catholics lie," etc., and these stereotypes are held by social groups without experience of their reality but of a shared personification of imagined peoples' behavior. The impact a cancer diagnosis has upon a patient is profound and complex for each patient brings to the diagnosis of cancer a worldview which has been constructed from early exposure to the term without any true knowledge of the illness. Therefore, the medical team must engage in both a debriefing of the false and erroneous ideas held by the misinformed patient as well as a re-education of the true nature of the disease.

The self-system is another dynamism which is crucial to personality structure. It functions as a security measure to protect the individual from anxiety (Sullivan, 1965). In order to avoid or minimize actual or potential anxiety, the person adopts various types of protective measures and supervisory controls over his behavior. These security measures form the self-system which sanctions certain forms of behavior, such as the "good-me" self, and forbids other forms of behavior, such as the "bad-me" self. We have found that this insight can be particularly helpful when dealing with a cancer patient who has a deep and irrational sense of personal guilt for having gotten the disease of cancer as if that patient has brought it upon himself as a "bad person." Handling the patient's sense of guilt is one of the great challenges in psychiatric oncology.

Sullivan's unique contribution to the role of cognition in personality theory has to do with his development of a threefold classification of experiences, for, says he, experiences occur in three different modes -- *protaxic, parataxic, and syntaxic.* These experiential modes merit a brief description of each in order to appreciate their relevance to Sullivan's understanding of interpersonal relations description of psychiatry. Sometimes called "types of experience" and sometimes called "types of cognition," this tripartite foundation of personality is worthy of close attention, owing to its relevance to the cancer patient's self-understanding and well-being.

The simplest and most fundamental mode of experiencing reality at the beginning of life is what Sullivan chose to call the *prototaxic* mode. It consists of essentially a flowing of sensations, feelings, and images without any necessary connection between them, a kind of "stream of consciousness," if you will. Sullivan himself describes it this way: "It may be regarded as the discrete series of momentary states of the sensitive organism" (1953). It occurs, of course, during the earliest months of infancy and must precede the others as a preparation for them. The *parataxic* mode of thinking, Sullivan explains, consists of seeing causal relationships between events that occur at about the same time but which are not logically related. Getting the connection wrong is what this mode of experience is all about. It is magical thinking, says he, for there is no logical connection between two events experienced by the child even though the child assumes there is. *Post hoc ergo propter hoc* is a concept in logical analysis which demonstrates a fallacy of reasoning by treating a sequence of unrelated events as relational in nature. For example, the prince of tea in China rises concurrently in time with the flooding of the Mississippi Rover – sequential but not causally related. It is essentially the "elementary externalization of causality." In childhood it occurs regularly when the child assumes that something he has done is the cause of something that is quite decidedly unrelated but he thinks it is. In adulthood, the residuals of parataxis modes of experiencing occur in such things as the presumed relationship between "praying hard" and "getting well." (See Appendix B for a discussion of the placebo effect of prayer.)

Finally, the third and most advanced mode of experience is called *syntaxic* and it corresponds to logical, analytical thought. *Syntaxic* experience of reality thus presupposes the ability to understand physical and spatial causality, and the ability to predict causes from knowledge of their effects. The meaning of words and the use of numbers constitutes the most poignant examples of the function of *syntaxic* experience and when the child learns the meaning of specific words and their uses and the nature of numbers and how they work, the child has reached this level of experiential sophistication needed in the development of interpersonal relationships. Reason and logic enter into the cognition of the individual such that scientific explanations may be grasped rationally thereby suspending superstition and magic as viable explanations of natural events. Understanding the nature of syntaxic experience can prove most valuable to the oncology team in treating patients.

Harry Stack Sullivan's distinctive contribution to contemporary psychiatry was his heavy emphasis upon the social factors which contribute to the development of human personality. Psychiatric oncology is the quintessential illustration of the confluence of biomedical psychiatry and psychosocial psychiatry embodied in the care and treatment of the cancer patient. Though schooled in Freudian psychoanalysis, he was not a Freudian in the sense that he differed from Freud in viewing the significance of the parent-child relationship as being an early quest for security rather than, as in Freudian psychoanalysis, primarily sexual in origin and nature. Drawing from his own personal life's story, Sullivan saw this child-mother relationship as central, not the sexual drive of libidinal instincts. Sullivan replaced Freud's drive theory of personality (libido driven) with his interpersonal theory of personality development (relationship drive). Sullivan, on the other hand, was intent upon integrating the multiple disciplines of the behavioral and social sciences into the work of psychiatry such that sociology and social psychology in the tradition of George Herbert Mead and Charles Horton Cooley proved most helpful in Sullivan's eventual development of what became known as *interpersonal psychiatry* and later *interpersonal psychotherapy* (Manis and Meltzer, 1972). He was not averse to reaching across disciplinary lines for theory and method, from evolution to communications, from learning theory to social organization. It was "interpersonal relations" which, he believed, constituted the fundamental ingredient in personality structure (Abraham and Morgan, 1989).

Sullivan's clinical work in a variety of settings over several years of medical assignments led him to firmly believe in the impact interpersonal relationships have upon personality development. He noted that individuals tend to carry distorted views and unrealistic expectations of others into their relationships. His solution was to become, as a clinical psychotherapist, a "participant observer" in dealing with his clients, taking a more active therapeutic stance than the traditional psychoanalytic "blank screen" approach popular at the time and particularly evident in the Freudian school of psychoanalysis (Freedheim, 1992). By focusing upon what he called "interpersonal behavior," he would observe the client's reaction to the therapist and the therapeutic environment. He believed that emotional well-being could be achieved by making an individual "aware" of their dysfunctional interpersonal patterns of interaction and thereby grow into a healthy self-awareness of their interactive behavior. This insight can prove most beneficial in psychiatric oncology's care of the patient as well (Morgan, 2020).

Sullivan's paradigmatic stages of personality development can be summed up in the expression, "everyone is much more simply human than otherwise." Having made this his standard operational modality, he utilized it throughout his career and summed up its meaning this way: "In other words, the differences between any two instances of human personality from the lowest grade imbecile to the highest grade genius -- are much less striking than the difference between the least gifted human being and a member of the nearest other biological genus." Sullivan was outspoken on this point (Sullivan, 1953; 1956; 1962). Denying that there were any real operative instincts left in the human person, and thus separating himself profoundly from Freud and the classical school of psychoanalysis, Sullivan contended that it is the social environment in which we mature that determines the effectiveness of our maturation. Interpersonal relationships are the essence of human development. We are only human in so far as we develop within the context of other people. We need to learn to compete, cooperate, and compromise with others as we mature in order to maintain mental health. "Personal individuality is an illusion," and therefore we exist only in relationship to other people according to Sullivan. When we mature within a healthy social environment, this positive progression of interpersonal events leads to an integrated personality, an adult who is capable of establishing satisfying interpersonal relations and who is able to both give and receive love. This is the essence of the human personality. Unfortunately and too often, the psychiatric oncologist is called upon to deal with personal and family dynamics which are less than healthy in the life of the patient and is, thus, left with a matrix of dysfunctional family relationships effectively stifling a healthy prognosis of social support.

Sullivan's elaborate and well developed description of the stages of human development was reminiscent of Freud's elaborate system. But, whereas Freud built his developmental scheme around the central core of childhood sexuality based on his drive theory of the libido, Sullivan's fundamental core of interpersonal relationships was based on developmental stages linked profoundly to the maturation of the personality. Sullivan's psychotherapeutic methodology was quite unique to his own understanding of the function and nature of interpersonal relationships. Sullivan firmly believed, based upon his extensive clinical experience, that mental disorders derive from interpersonal failures rather than a biochemical imbalance as promoted by Kraepelin (Morgan, 2020) and, therefore, therapeutic procedures must be based upon a genuine effort to improve the patient's relationship skills in dealing with others. In keeping with his overall worldview, interpersonal relationships constitute the core of psychotherapeutic treatment. In this situation, it is imperative that the therapist understand that his role is primarily that of a "participant observer," for, despite all protestations to the contrary from traditionalists, the therapist becomes necessarily part of an interpersonal, face-to-face relationship with the patient.

This process actually creates the opportunity for the patient to establish a syntaxic communication with another person, namely, the therapist himself. The central relevance of this insight must also be embraced by the medical team in dealing with the cancer patient.

Because of the emphasis upon the therapeutic role being that of an "observer," the therapist is exempt from becoming "involved" with the patient but, as with the Freudian tradition, the therapist must establish a relationship based upon his role as an expert in relationships, instead of as a friend, chum, or colleague. Unlike the work of Carl Rogers in client-centered therapy (Rogers, 1970; Morgan, 2017), Sullivan is insistent that the therapist "not" become a friend of the patient, thereby destroying the "observational" character of the therapist's relationship to the patient. Sullivan had three primary objectives in the therapeutic situation. The practical utility of this insight can be of great benefit to the oncology team in dealing with the terminal patient. First, he intends to help the patient improve foresight, discover difficulties in interpersonal relations, and restore the ability to participate in consensually validated experiences. This occurs when three questions are addressed: "(1) How can I best put into words what I wish to say to the patient? (2) What is the general pattern of communication between us? and (3) What precisely is the patient saying to me?" These are not simplistic?

In some circles, Harry Stack Sullivan is considered the "father of modern psychiatry," but, of course, this consideration pre-dates the emergence of the psychiatrist as a "medication monitor"! Today, unlike in Sullivan's own day, psychiatry has been disastrously reduced to monitoring medication without the slightest effort to offer therapeutic counseling which has, by and large, been left to either the social worker or the pastoral counselor. Psychiatry can no longer function as the therapeutic dispenser it was from Freud to Sullivan because the insurance companies and the HMOs have precluded the affordability of such practice (Morgan, 2020). Psychiatrist must dispense and monitor the psychopharmacological industry's involvement with clients and patients, leaving whatever counseling might be called for to other professionals, namely, social workers and pastoral counselors. Of course, it is the patient and client who suffer, but such is the fee-driven market system operative in American society today. Herein rests the challenge to a responsive oncology team concerned not just with the medical side of cancer treatment but the psychosocial matrix of the holistic health care of the patient as well.

CHAPTER FIVE
THE EMOTIONAL SPECTRUM OF A TERMINAL DIAGNOSIS

Addressing the Psychosocial Issues in Psychiatric Oncology

The psychopathology of end of life issues continues to expand relative to the insights provided by psychotherapeutic counseling within the framework of *psychiatric oncology*. Death from cancer constitutes a special category of terminal health studies owing to the specificity of that diagnosis, a descriptive designation fraught with ambiguity, confusion, and even anger on the part of both the patient and the family involved. The issues are both simple and complex; simple in the sense that the end of life is the inevitability of a terminal diagnosis and complex in terms of how both the patient and the family handle such reality. It is the rare individual for whom the simple platitudinous answers provided by religion are sufficient to ward off fear, anxiety, and depression. For everyone else in search of a meaningful acknowledgment of this reality such that it might be dealt with rationally and responsibly, more is and should be demanded by the patient. The following enquiry covers a broad spectrum of psychological and emotional issues confronting both the terminal patient and the family involved in the care of that patient. This enquiry is decidedly not a how-to effort on how to deal with the subject but rather a collection of insightful investigations addressing analytically a range of situations, attitudes, emotions, and practical issues that affect and are affected by both the patient and the family. Finally, it needs to be said plainly here that we are dealing specifically with the psychological and social aspects of the phenomenon of the terminal cancer patient and not with the medical complexities of the illness. The oncological care of the cancer patient rests with the medical personnel while the psychosocial issues are dealt with by a trained psychopathologist. It is the psychiatric oncologist who embraces both agendas.

The labeling of this approach to the study of an emotional behavioral matrix produced by an oncological diagnosis early constituted, if not a controversy, at least an initial stage of ambiguity. Relevant here is Alfred Adler's experience of naming his new approach to psychotherapy *individual psychology* following the rather distinguished term of *psychoanalysis* developed by Freud (Adler, 1927; Hoffman, 1994). Then, there was Carl Jung who chose the rather bland and non-descriptive term *analytical psychology* for his lame attempt at competing Freud. Viktor Frankl faced the same practical issue in the naming of *logotherapy*, initially preferring *existential analysis* which had, alas, already been taken (Frankl, 1946).. The task and agenda of psychiatric oncology has been from the beginning quite clear, namely, to address the psychosocial issues involved in a diagnosis of cancer within the framework of the medical diagnosis. The clinically systematic analysis and assessment of the psychological, behavioral, emotional and social issues which occur as a result of a diagnosis of cancer for both the patient and the involved family constituted the matrix of research and study brought forth by psychiatric oncologists at the Sloan Kettering Cancer Center in New York in the early 1970s. The regrettable mishap in naming this approach "psycho-oncology" is only the result of a *zeitgeist* attitude that anything not considered as normal behavior is "psycho," alas even Hollywood named a leading movie such. Moving beyond that misstep in nomenclature, the term *psychosocial oncology* took early precedence over *psychiatric oncology* preferring to avoid the false impression that its research agenda is in some way a manifestation of medical psychiatry. Since this sub-discipline is not medical but psychological, sociological, emotional and behavioral, the focus of research is two-fold, namely, addressing the emotional state of the patient diagnosed with cancer as well as addressing the emotional and behavioral issues arising from within the matrix of the patient/family dynamic which results from the diagnosis.

Clearly, psychiatric oncology received a great boost in credibility as a viable research and training specialization when the Memorial Sloan Kettering Cancer Center (MSKCC) authenticated the efforts in this new and exciting adventure. The MSKCC is one of the most respected cancer research and training institutions in the United States. Founded in 1884 in New York City, it eventually received a substantial gift from General Motors and subsequently adopted the combined names of the president, Alfred P. Sloan, and vice president, Charles F. Kettering, of General Motors. It was within this institutional setting where Dr. Jimmie Holland commenced her historic work in the study of emotional factors involved in the treatment of cancer patients and the rise of the specialization in psychiatric oncology has continued its rise as a leading orientation in the care of terminal cancer patients and their families.

Within the context of the medical specialization of cancer care, psychiatric oncology was granted a unique opportunity to demonstrate the need for and effectiveness of the emotional and behavioral care of the patients and their families facing a terminal diagnosis as well as the need for the training of the professional caregivers within this setting. Embracing the viability of concerns for the intersection of the psychological, social, and behavioral characteristics of terminal cancer encountered by the patient and the patient's family, the professional staff of the Sloan-Kettering Clinic was clearly cognizant of the need for the effective training of the attending personnel based on the emotional complexities of the diagnostic event. From diagnosis through the treatment regime to its final conclusion involving end-of-life issues and subsequent survivor needs, the reality of the terminal cancer patient's knowledge regarding the diagnosis as well as that of the involved family was held in constant awareness by the caregivers (Holland and Bultz, 2007; Holland, 1986, 2002).

The emotional spectrum covered in the case of a terminal diagnosis of cancer covers a broad range of psychological and behavioral as well as social manifestations not specifically found within other diagnoses of acute medical exigencies (Zabora et al, 2001; Carlson et al, 2004). From the initial patient reaction to the diagnosis to the family's response to the reality of a terminal condition, there is a litany of emotionally-charged reactions ranging from elevated states of depression and anxiety to practical physiological responses linked to a shift in body consciousness and self-image. The psychiatric oncologist at the Sloan Kettering Cancer Center is trained to identify and to attempt to mitigate the negative ground-swell of emotions which often accompanies the diagnosis. However, clinical cases have surprisingly demonstrated in some instances the patient actually experiencing an elevation of an emotional sense of well-being.

A cancer diagnosis most commonly precipitates and not infrequently exacerbates manifestations of acute depression and anxiety, often reaching debilitating and occasionally suicidal levels of intensity. Such a diagnosis often includes overriding concerns regarding the treatment protocols themselves such as hair loss, nausea, fatigue, pain, and something commonly called "chemo-brain" (real or imagined). The trained psychiatric oncologist, most often a clinically trained psychopathologist with a Ph.D. or Psy.D. (rather than an M.D.), is equipped to identify and respond to these potentially debilitating reactions to the diagnosis (Derogatis et al, 1983).

The overriding issue and resulting agenda for the attending professional staff as well as the patient and family involves the quality of life especially as linked to shorter survival issues characterizing the patient and the long-term issues related to the survivors (Petticrew, Bell, Hunter, 2002). Roth and Cohen (1986) have called attention to two types of "coping" mechanisms on the part of the patient, a positive and a negative composite of relevant behavioral and emotionally-charged responses to the terminal diagnosis.

There is what is called the *approach coping* mechanism wherein the patient takes on a positive, even energetic, attitude regarding the diagnosis and commences to embrace a positive and pro-active stance involving both the patient's own attitudes and the call by the patient for the family and support group to do likewise. The negative response is called *avoidance coping* and reflects a negative attitude and response on the part of the patient and commonly the family support group as well. The characteristics of this negativity include a disinclination to discuss the reality of the terminal diagnosis with the professional staff or family members.

Thanks to the work of Stanton and colleagues (2002), they have identified a behavioral response nurtured by the psychiatric oncologist within the patient called *benefit finding* which is essentially a self-reflective matrix of behavior designed to seek out and identify opportunities for a positive participation in the diagnostic and treatment protocol such that the patient identifies more as an assisting participant in their own treatment process rather than merely the subject of the treatment. Benefit finding often precipitates an effective coping strategy wherein the patient is called upon and has the opportunity of assessing the meaning and scope of one's own life in which an evaluative posture may be developed proving effective in staving off depression and anxiety. Researchers such as Barskova and

Oesterreich (2009) have shown that what they have chosen to call *post-traumatic growth* can prove profoundly helpful to self-reflective patients who have determined to assess the meaning of their life situation including the inevitability of mortality and what an existential embrace of the moment might offer in the midst of the terminal diagnosis. Such efforts, according to Lee (2008) has shown to prove beneficial to the patient who can move beyond the initial trauma of diagnosis to a post-traumatic growth posture embracing the inevitability of a limited future. Such quality of life issues, though often sounding trite, can provide a solid basis upon which the psychiatric oncologist can maneuver the patient to a stronger footing in facing the uncertainties of the future.

Two significant components of the overall pattern of care for the patient overseen by the psychiatric oncologist is that of compliance with treatment protocols on the part of the patient immediately commenced at the time of receiving the cancer diagnosis. Recognition of the central importance of the social support network available to the patient is crucial for the implementation of a healthy treatment protocol. In the past the dominant role in cancer treatment rested exclusively or primarily with the attending medical team with the patient somewhat reduced to a passively receptive posture. In recent years the relationship between the health provider and the recipient has approached parity in terms of compliance to treatment protocol responsibilities wherein the patient is called upon to be more directly and actively involved in treatment. The team of DiMatteo, Lepper and Croghan (2000) has clinically demonstrated the effectiveness of fostering this sense of shared responsibility and collaborative protocol compliance resulting in a more meaningful participatory role on the part of the patient. Greer and colleagues (2016) have shown that this emphasis upon collaborative compliance to treatment protocols is particularly helpful at the commencement of chemotherapy and the resulting demands on the patient for conscientious adherence to guideline directives. Such studies are beginning to demonstrate that depression and anxiety are both reduced when this shared collaboration is employed.

Though Valtorta and colleagues (2016) have clinical evidence showing that patients suffering from cardiovascular disease benefit significantly from a strong social network of support, Nausheen and his team (2009) have shown clinical evidence of this kind of network support being of particular significance and benefit to terminally diagnosed cancer patients. This matrix of support from the oncology team proves relevant to both the patient as well as to the family who themselves are faced with the uncertainties and complications of medical expense, care of children, insurance issues, property care and maintenance, etc., not to mention the anticipated physical impairments resulting from chemotherapy and cognate medical procedures. Holt-Lunstad and collaborative researchers (2015) have clinical evidence demonstrating that the negative impact of both physical and emotional diminishment radically affects the patient as well as the family's attitudes about the future with Greer and colleagues (2010) showing that the oncology team employing Cognitive Behavior Therapy (CBT) proves frequently beneficial in intervention related patient depression.

Throughout the considerable engagement necessitated in treatment between the patient and the care team, meaningful communication consistently has proven to be a determining factor in the effective management of the patient's sense of well-being. Zolnierek and DiMatteo (2009) as well as Waldron and colleagues (2013) have provided clinically demonstrative evidence specifically illustrating this effect. Santosh K. Chaturvedi has provided a particularly detailed and elaborate recitation of the complexities of cancer care to which psychiatric oncology has demonstrated a profoundly effective capability. His work (1994) centered upon a longitudinal study in India where he was former Dean of the Behavioral Sciences and Senior Professor of Psychiatry in the National Institute of

Mental Health and Neurosciences. His study has proven to be a standard-bearer in validating the efficacy of the psychosocial approach to oncology treatment as a companion protocol to the medical demands brought by a terminal diagnosis of cancer (Chaturvedi and Chandra, 2010).

The fundamental challenge, however, from the beginning of this specialization has been the cost of services. As modern psychiatry moved away from psychotherapeutic counseling and began embracing psychopharmacology due to the expense variant from that of the clinical hour to the medication option, so likewise the oncology community has had to deal with the realities of cost of services. Psychiatry in both training and practice has moved decidedly away from psychotherapy and towards medication as the most effective response to mental illness when costs and time factors are considered. The shift from a focus upon causal factors in psychiatric care and towards behavior modification has become the dominant protocol in modern psychiatry. A clinical hour is costly and restricts the number of patients the psychiatrist can see on a daily basis. Whereas psychotherapy can accommodate five or six patients per day at 50 minute intervals, psychopharmacological psychiatry can accommodate five times that many patients per day and, from the patient's point of view, much less expensive in terms of both cost and time requirements. Of course, medication does cost but counseling runs commonly above $150.00 a clinical hour whereas many antidepressants cost mere pennies (Morgan, 2021). Clearly, from causation to behavior modification in the treatment of mental disorders is now the standard operating procedure.

The questions, both professional and ethical, come to the psychiatrist in the form of what quality of care can be given the patient and at what expense to the psychiatrist (as well as to the patient), keeping in mind that insurance companies as well as public health services are extremely conservative in terms of supporting mental health care. Psychotherapy is usually outside standard coverage whereas mediations are more commonly covered. Likewise, psychiatric oncology faces just these very same issues, namely, how expensive are such services for the attending medical staff and institution as against the benefits experienced by the patient (Syrjala et al, 2014). Addressing the emotional spectrum of a cancer diagnosis with therapeutic counseling where depression and anxiety are the presenting issues as well as the requirements of time consumed by both patient and psychiatrist versus a medication prescription for depression and anxiety without any time requirements seems to weigh heavily upon the practicalities of choice between psychotherapy and medication (Osborn, Demoncada, and Feuerstein, 2006).

As is commonly known, serotonin reuptake inhibitors have proven very effective in the treatment of depression and anxiety as well as the more well-known drugs including benzodiazepines. The reality is the behavioral characteristics of depression and anxiety are effectively addressed with such medication. The down side, however, is the causality of depression is not addressed by medication whereas psychotherapy addresses specifically the psychological causes of depression and has been clinically shown to be very effective (Morgan, 2020, 2021). What seems to be called for here is a collaborative effort of both psychotherapy and medication, a holistic team approach involving psychotherapy and psychopharmacology all under the overall purview of the attending oncologist. (See Appendix B "Medication and Counseling").

Balancing concerns for the emotional well-being of the terminal cancer patient and the family involved where psychotherapeutic assistance is clearly called for against the practicalities of medical staff time and expense, what might then be the practical utility of psychiatric oncology within the clinical setting or hospital? At one level, such a service is simply not practical in terms of cost and staff time and, therefore, consideration of the benefits of psychiatric oncology must necessarily be weighed against sound medical oncological practice coupled, when needed, with psychopharmacological assistance or intervention. And yet, might something of relevance to the attending oncologists' knowledge and care of the patient be gained from a closer examination of the psychosocial issues involved in a terminal diagnosis? When to prescribe an anti-depressant medication and when to recommend (and even provide?) psychotherapeutic counseling might not be out of bounds for the primary care givers' consideration (Waldron et al, 2013). Keeping in mind that the psychosocial issues involving a terminally ill cancer patient are comprehensively palliative rather curative, the existential care for the patient and the long-term assistance to the survivors seem not to be outside the spectrum of good medical practice. The bold issue for any medical practice is, of course and always will be, how the hosting institution is able to justify the non-remunerative expense involved in providing such a holistic package of psychotherapy and psychopharmacology administered by the oncological team. When both the public health services and the standard-level medical insurance industry are resistant to such care, from where is funding to be had for such care (Morgan, 2015)?

Nevertheless, the gradual but inevitable recognition within the medical community of the importance of addressing the emotional needs of the terminally diagnosed patient has over the years produced a response of creative developments within patient care such as is illustrated in the work of the Sloan-Kettering Clinic. When professionals trained in psychopathology collaborate with medical specialists in oncology in the overall care of the terminal patient, clinical evidence proves that everyone benefits – patient, family, staff. The fact that oncology clinics are beginning to put on staff psychologists specializing in psychiatric oncology suggests a growing cognizance of this more inclusive holistic approach to the care and treatment of the terminally diagnosed cancer patient. Much research and study remains to be done covering a broad spectrum of issues but with a deepening awareness of the effectively productive collaboration between the medical and the behavioral science communities, the future is full of promise.

CHAPTER SIX
A RANGE OF SPECIALIZED PROGRAMS IN PSYCHIATRIC ONCOLOGY

Leading Medical Institutions in the United States

As has been pointed out and discussed earlier, the labeling of this specialization has caused some confusion and not a little controversy within the medical community both from the perspective of oncology itself and from within the psychiatric and psychotherapeutic communities as well. This issue is not soon to disappear, if it ever does, for each of the various institutional implementation of this specialization have made such an investment in its development that to reach a consensus throughout the medical community seems most unlikely. What has been done in the following discussion is a brief summary overview of several of the leading cancer treatment centers in the U.S. which have set the standard for the psychosocial treatment of the cancer patient. Within each institution a specialized nomenclature has been adopted to characterize its own particular perspective in both theory and practice. At the end of the day, however, it will become clear that even though there is a variance in the labeling of this specialization, the overall character of the theory and practice is so very similar that the only significant variation seems to be in the labeling itself rather than the modality of treatment, whether it be psycho-oncology, psychosocial oncology, psych-oncology, or psychiatric oncology.

AMERICAN PSYCHO-ONCOLOGY SOCIETY (APOS)

Before we launch an institutional overview of nationally recognized programs and services, it should be pointed out that the American Psycho-Oncology Society (APOS), which was founded in 1986, promotes psychosocial oncology as a cancer specialty designed to address a full range of issues in the psychological, behavioral, emotional, and social spectrum of cancer treatment care of both the patient and the family. This professional body of over 2,000 members has been formed to focus a high-level of professional awareness of and response to the dynamics of emotional factors affecting the cancer patient and the community beyond those of the bio-medical care and treatment of cancer. The APOS calls attention to such issues as the relevance of the type of cancer involved in patient care, age and life situation of the patient and supporting family, and coping mechanisms present and absent in the family's matrix of care. Promoting psychosocial oncology as that specialization within oncological patient care which focuses upon the behavioral and emotional spectrum of affective issue, this professional body is fully cognizant of the fact that whatever the label employed by an institution of care and professional body of interest, whether psychosocial oncology, psycho-oncology, psych-oncology, or psychiatric oncology, they are all designed to address issues of emotional and behavioral care of the cancer patient within the context of a medical institution and medical team of professionals trained in a confluence of biomedical specializations as well as psychosocial specializations. The APOS is the only organization within this discussion which lists chaplains as part of the health care team along with social workers, psychologists, psychiatrists, nurses, and mental health counselors. The APOS recognizes that even though the religious orientation of the cancer patient and supporting family may prove to constitute a functional placebo for a compassionate God, the medical team is oriented towards the science of biomedical and psychosocial care without presuming to promote a belief-system or faith-based understanding of cancer care without challenging the patient's own religious ideologies. While holding in check the danger of an over-reach by the clergy into the arena of medical science, the support team is fully aware of the emotional support which a religious orientation may provide to the patient involved in a religious worldview. Prayer and notions of Divine Intervention, though standing clearly outside the scientific matrix of medical care, may be called upon by the religious patient and family where there is a faith-based tradition. (This has been considered in Appendix A).

ONCOLOGY NURSING SOCIETY (ONS)

The Oncology Nursing Society (ONS) is institutionally connected to the Sloan-Kettering Cancer Center which was founded by Jimmie Holland, M.D., the Oncology Nursing Society with its 35,000 membership is not directly linked to a particular medical center or hospital and while standing upon its own foundation, ONS is not in competition with or at odds with the philosophy of the American Psycho-Oncology Society. Rather, it traces its origins to 1973 and the first National Cancer Nursing Research Conference which was sponsored by the American Nurses Association and the American Cancer Society. In the following consideration of several leading medical institutions embodying the concept of psychiatric oncology, we will find that many of their nursing staff employees are active members of the Oncology Nursing Society. A distinctive feature of ONS is its active involvement in advocacy issues related to cancer patient care at the local, state, and national levels, hosting annually the largest conference of oncology nursing professionals in the world.

The Society represents a broad spectrum of professional specializations including registered nurses, advanced practice nurses, case managers, researchers and healthcare professional educators. To further develop and enhance the professional level of its membership, the Society offers accredited continuing nursing educational programs, both online and residential, endorsed by the American Nurses Credentialing Center's Commission on Accreditation. It maintains two internationally recognized scholarly periodicals, the *Oncology Nursing Forum* and the *Clinical Journal of Oncology Nursing* as well as the Society's news magazine, *ONS Voice.* Combined with an aggressive publishing agenda in books, guidelines, and standards of cancer care, ONS has secured its role as the leader in oncology nursing education.

One outstanding feature of the Oncology Nursing Society's website is their generous listing of international professional bodies of nurses which we list here taken from their website:

National nursing organizations

The Trained Nurses' Association of India

United Nurses Association (India)

Alliance of Young Nurse Leaders and Advocates

American Nurses Association

An Board Altranais

Canadian Indigenous Nurses Association

Canadian Nurses Association

Japanese Nursing Association

Nursing Council of Kenya (Nursing in Kenya)

Nursing Association of Nepal

Indian nurses association (India)

Nursing Council of New Zealand

Nursing and Midwifery Council

New Zealand Nurses Organisation

Philippine Nurses Association

Philippine Nurses Association of United Kingdom

Nursing & Midwifery Council United

Certification and accreditation boards

Bangladesh Nursing and Midwifery Council (BNMC)

American Nurses Credentialing Center (ANCC)

National Certification Corporation (NCC)

National Council of State Boards of Nursing

National League for Nursing Accrediting Commission (NLNAC)

Indian Nursing Council (see also state nursing councils in India)

Honor societies

Sigma Theta Tau International Honor Society of Nursing

Professional Fraternities

Alpha Tau Delta (collegiate, professional fraternity in nursing)

Chi Eta Phi (collegiate, predominantly African-American professional sorority in nursing)

Specialty organizations

Academy of Medical-Surgical Nurses (AMSN)

Academy of Neonatal Nursing

American Academy of Nurse Practitioners

American Association of Legal Nurse Consultants

American Association of Nurse Anesthetists

American College of Nurse Practitioners

American Psychiatric Nurses Association

Association of Nurses in AIDS Care

Association of PeriOperative Registered Nurses

Association of Women's Health, Obstetric and Neonatal Nurses (AWHONN)

NANDA

National Black Nurses Association

Society of Gynecologic Nurse Oncologists

Space Nursing Society

Unions

Australian Nursing Federation

Canadian Federation of Nurses' Union

California Nurses Association/National Nurses Organizing Committee (CNA/NNOC)

Democratic Nursing Organisation of South Africa

Finnish Union of Practical Nurses

Manitoba Nurses' Union

National Nurses United (NNU)

New South Wales Nurses and Midwives' Association

New Zealand Nurses Organisation

Pennsylvania Association of Staff Nurses and Allied Professionals

Queensland Nurses' Union

Royal College of Nursing

South African Democratic Nurses' Union

Tennessee Nurses Association

United American Nurses

United Nurses of Alberta

Washington State Nurses Association

Miscellaneous

American Academy of Nursing

American Association of Colleges of Nursing

American Health Care Association

American Red Cross Nursing Service

Florence Network for Nursing and Midwifery

International Council of Nurses

National Institute of Nursing Research

National League for Nursing (NLN)

Nursing Students Without Borders

National Student Nurses' Association (U.S.)

Registered Nurses' Association of Ontario

INDIANA UNIVERSITY SCHOOL OF MEDICINE

In making the appointment announcement of the first "Walther Scholar in Psycho-Oncology," the Indiana University School of Medicine chose to speak of "supportive oncology" in the April 26, 2022, news release wherein the article emphasized that in the Medical School's standard therapeutic treatments of cancer using surgery, chemotherapy and radiation, attention was called to the further efforts to attend to the patient's overall "physical, mental and spiritual well-being." Throughout the medical community both the physical and mental health of the cancer patient is recognized and addressed but the use of the undefined term "spiritual well-being" has from the beginning constituted a point of concern, anxiety, and controversy throughout medical practice. The IU Program in psycho-oncology has been designed specifically to attend to the needs of the "underserved." The newly appointed director emphasizes the Walther Cancer Foundation's support which is designed to address the fundamental issues confronted by individuals and families whose lives have been challenged by cancer with special attention to clinical studies focusing upon "mind-body interventions" in quest of nurturing both "physical health and psychological well-being" of the patient. From the announcement, it appears that the IU Medical School is using interchangeably the terms "spiritual well-being" and "psychological well-being" and if such is the case then the anxieties raised by the use of the term "spiritual" are somewhat allayed. Because the Indiana University School of Medicine is a state-funded and governed entity, clarification of the distinction between the terms "spiritual" and "psychological" would be most helpful but, as with most medical institutions, there is an orchestrated effort to avoid definitional distinctions in deference to laws related to church and state (religion and secular) issues.

DANA-FARBER CANCER INSTITUTE

The Department of Adult Psychosocial Oncology and Palliative Care at the Dana-Farber Cancer Institute is headed by Ilana Braun, M.D. This research and treatment institution is recognized as the founding member of the Dana-Farber/Harvard Cancer Center at Harvard University's comprehensive cancer center. Acknowledged internationally as the third ranked cancer hospital in the world, this Cancer Institute has chosen to label its emotional care of cancer patients "psychosocial oncology" rather than psycho-oncology, focusing its clinical efforts in adult palliative care and adult social work as well as pediatric psychosocial oncology. The departmental orientation combines psychosocial oncology and palliative care targeting the development of an individual treatment plan designed to help the patient (and family) deal with what it terms "emotional stress" through the developmental stages of cancer progression consisting of "anxiety and sadness, depression, family coping, relationship issues, personal, spiritual and existential issues, and changes in thinking and behavior." Again, as with the Indiana University Medical School, the use of the word "spiritual" is employed when speaking of the emotional well-being of the patient (and family). The Dana-Farber medical team consists of medical oncologists, nurses trained in cancer care, and a supportive care team of clinical physicians, psychologists, social workers, and pharmacologists providing palliative care for the patient dealing with pain "and other physical, emotional, and spiritual distress" during illness and end of life issues.

THE HELEN DILLER CANCER CENTER/UNIVERSITY OF CALIFORNIA

The Helen Diller Cancer Center (HDCC) at the University of California in San Francisco has opted for the term psycho-oncology but has chosen to mention "Spiritual Care Services" only briefly in their listing of a roster of collaborative support programs such as their Patient and Family Cancer Support Center, Social Work, Spiritual care Services, Art for Recovery, the Osher Center for Integrative Medicine and the Symptom Management Service programs which have been developed by the University Hospital to address the broad spectrum of emotional needs of both the patient and the family. The overall emphasis promoted by the Center is embodied in the work of psychologists and psychiatrists specifically trained in dealing with behavioral issues affecting patient morale, treatment and survivorship issues. Concerns over pain, insomnia, eating challenges and emotional issues are integrated into a broad-based spectrum of treatment modalities. A particularly strong emphasis in this range of response treatments emphasizes survivorship wellness group programs consisting of stress management skills, cognitive behavioral therapy, mindfulness, acceptance and commitment therapy, and cancer survivorship health strategies, this latter being one which is commonly underemphasized in many cancer care institutions but is intentionally elevated at the Diller Cancer Center as a key feature.

CENTER FOR PSYCHIATRIC ONCOLOGY AND BEHAVAIORAL SCIENCES (MASSACHUSETTS GENERAL HOSPITAL IN BOSTON)

One of the most important and internationally acclaimed medical institutions which has embraced the emotional side of cancer care is that of the Center for Psychiatric Oncology and Behavioral Sciences at Massachusetts General Hospital in Boston. From its very beginning, the Center promoted the collaborative relationship between psychiatry and psychology in its efforts to focus attention upon the whole patient rather than differentiating between the biomedical approach and the psychosocial approach to patient care. In their presentation of the Center's mission, Mass General makes the point that individuals with severe mental illness die nearly 25 years earlier than the general population and many of those deaths are attributed to cancer. This constituted the focus and mission of the Center, to address the mental health of the cancer patient in an attempt to up the quality of life of the terminal individual suffering from cancer. This Center was among the first major medical institutions in the U.S. to employ the term "psychiatric oncology" to characterize their approach and perspective. And, in order to provide a cognitive bridge with those specifically involved in the emotional side of cancer care, the Center added "Behavioral Sciences" to their formal name.

It is the whole patient they wish to treat and not to conspicuously differentiate the medical from the emotional. Recognizing that there is inevitably an extreme stress upon the individual diagnosed with cancer in terms of emotional well-being, the Department of Psychiatry and the Cancer Center have joined together to address these issues including not just the emotional care of the patient but of the family involved as well. Thanks to the continuing support of the National Cancer Institute, the Center for Psychiatric Oncology and Behavioral Sciences at Mass General has identified seven specific areas of research and treatment, viz., depression, anxiety, survivorship, access to care, disparities, aging, and health behaviors. Each area is researched from a confluence of both biomedical and psychosocial clinical perspectives. Owing to this collaborative approach to holistic care, the Cancer Center at

Mass General is able, with precession, to distinguish between treatment modalities focusing upon specifically those behavioral and emotional issues confronting the patient as well as those bio-physiological issues which inevitably present potential points of stress and anxiety in the patient. These include nutritional concerns, metastasis, chemotherapy, and radiotherapy changes resulting from treatment. Within the matrix of this diagnostic challenge, the Center is able to construct a treatment plan which is responsive to the inevitable adjustments resulting from a diagnostic assess and disease-related physical changes produced by such variables as age, gender, personality, background and beliefs.

A fundamental characteristic of the Mass General Cancer Center treatment protocol is that every patient is cared for by a collaborative multidisciplinary team of medical professionals specializing in psychiatric oncology. This protocol approach developed by the Cancer Center at Mass General includes the active participation of select family members, the referring physician, and the oncology team of both medical and psychiatric oncologists with special care paid to issues related to patient anxiety, patient participatory involvement in treatment protocols, medication adjustments and the inevitable psychological aspects of cancer affecting both patient and family.

Owing to the expense of training and time factors affecting medical performance of personnel, many medical facilities find it financially prohibitive to provide trained psychiatric oncology professionals. This Caner Center prides itself on always providing a comprehensive psychiatric evaluation of every cancer patient by both psychiatrists and oncologists who have undergone specific psychiatric training in the emotional care of cancer patients thereby providing a coalescence of both medical and psychological insights and understanding of patient distress and anxiety. Given the breadth of training of the psychiatric oncology staff, issues related to psychotropic medications sometimes called for in the treatment of the cancer patient under severe stress and anxiety is coupled with access to counseling and psychotherapeutic intervention including the full cooperation of the Oncology Social Work and Behavioral Medicine Services provided by the Cancer Center.

A major feature of a research hospital is the involvement of its medical staff in on-going research directly related to the clinical studies being conducted within the institution itself. Mass General leads the country as one of the major such medical centers and the patients being served are always the ultimate beneficiaries of such research-oriented medical team collaboration. The three major areas of focused institutional research are depression, anxiety, and health behaviors. All three fall conveniently into both biomedical and psychosocial oncology matrices of care and treatment. An example of their clinical study of depression focuses upon the relationship between types of chemotherapy and the elevation of depression compared to reported fatigue rather than depression. On-going clinical studies of anxiety are providing insights into the relationship of treatment and completion protocols and the prospects of behavioral intervention providing therapeutic effectiveness in advanced lung cancer patients. One major challenging study currently underway in health behavior studies involves the relationship of insurance coverage and smoking and ways in which pharmacological intervention for smokers may prove efficacious in the cessation or diminishment of habitual smoking behavior and the eventuality of cancer.

MD ANDERSON PSYCHIATRIC ONCOLOGY CENTER

The MD Anderson Psychiatric Oncology Center in Houston, Texas, has chosen to join other internationally recognized medical research institutions in adopting the term "psychiatric oncology" rather than the other labeling options such as psychosocial oncology, psycho-oncology, and psych-oncology. Their psychiatric emphasis centers around symptom assessment and medical management, stress management, cognitive behavior therapy, sexual counseling, substance abuse assessment, referral and follow-up, therapy for families, couples, children and adolescents, and a general support group for caregivers. The Center has a special emphasis upon the important of providing emotional support for those professionals directly involved in providing care for the cancer patient and family members. This emphasis is indicative of the Center's recognition of the central importance of the medical care team as major contributors to the enhancement of patient care generated from within the ranks of the health care team itself. By taking care of the care givers, the care receivers will all benefit. This constitutes the operational approach to the functioning of the MD Anderson Psychiatric Oncology Center.

UNIVERSITY OF MICHIGAN ROGEL CANCER CENTER

Following its own best insights into the nature and function of this specialization within oncology, the University of Michigan Rogel Cancer Center has chosen the rather unique label for its efforts called "PsychOncology" thereby attempting to avoid the dangers of a misperception of what in the minds of the general public is mistakenly linked to the word "psycho" as if the "psycho" in the term "psycho-oncology" had to do with mental illness, i.e., the mentally ill cancer patient. The RCC attempts to avoid both the overly medical-sounding "psychiatric oncology" as well as the overly psychologically-sounding "psychosocial oncology." The argument goes on without end but the Rogel Cancer Center has distinguished itself in its efforts on the part of the patient to relieve the "numerous negative social and psychological effects of the disease." A particular feature of their overall program draws from an educational agenda offered to the patient and family regarding issues related to the emotional dynamics of a cancer diagnosis. Such educational programs are hosted at the Cancer Center and cover such relevant topics as parenting with cancer, grief and loss issues and how to handle the holidays within the context of cancer. In dealing with stress and depression issues within the patient as well as the family, such topics as feelings of guilt and anger resulting from the diagnosis are considered within the context of self-image and quality of life issues confronting both patient and family. Staffing of the Center draws from various hospital departments addressing both the biomedical side of cancer as well as the emotional psychodynamic side. The PsychOncology program covers educational and counseling assistance as well as what they characterize as "social, emotional, and spiritual needs" of the patient (but without an attempt to define the parameters of the term "spiritual" though chaplaincy is never mentioned.) Specialists mentioned in their descriptive literature include social workers, psychiatrists, psychologists, child and family life therapists, nurses, art therapists and what they label as "complementary therapy professionals." Some within the profession have suggested that the Rogel Cancer Center has come closer in its labeling of their program as PsychOncology than has any of the other terms such as psycho-oncology and psychosocial oncology excepting the more traditional medically-oriented term of psychiatric oncology.

CHAPTER SEVEN
A CROSS-CULTURAL APPROACH TO PSYCHIATRIC ONCOLOGY

Consultation Liaison Psychiatry in Review

The following summary is of a paper by Santosh K. Chaturvedi, M.D., given at the Annual National Conference of the Indian Psychiatric Society in 2012. The essay constitutes an interfacing of psychiatric oncology and Consultation Liaison Psychiatry. (The bibliographic source for this article is in the *Indian Journal of Psychiatry*. 2012 April-June; 54(2): 111-118.)

The author of over 600 articles in the field of psychiatry, Dr. Santosh K. Chaturvedi is one of the most recognized medical research scholars in the world and has led the work done in psychiatry in India for decades. An early proponent of psychiatric oncology, Dr. Chaturvedi has contributed a broadened understanding of this specialization within oncological research and treatment by the introduction and development of what he has chosen to call Consultation Liaison Psychiatry (CLP). In this overview article there is a specific focus upon the work being done in India in the field of psychiatry oncology. At the time of his lecture reviewed here, psychiatric oncology was gaining international attention and Chaturvedi was among the first in India to see the profound benefits in its approach to a holistic treatment of cancer patients. Though quick to credit Dr. Jimmie Holland for her early work at the Sloan Kettering Cancer Center where Chaturvedi first met and worked with Dr. Holland and her team, it must be kept in mind that the pioneering work done in India in the early days of the development of psychiatric oncology was in the hands and under the leadership of Chaturvedi himself.

Recognizing that psychiatric oncology was effective in identifying psychosocial components of health and healing within the oncological community, Indian researchers commenced the extension of this overall approach under the leadership of Chaturvedi to develop a systemic approach they chose to label Consultation Liaison Psychiatry (CLP). This broad-based approach to cancer care and treatment includes clinical studies of pain and palliative care and the screening for psychiatric morbidity as well as a careful look at the quality of life issues being faced by cancer patients. The development of communication skills among the care givers constitutes a focus of CLP as well as the emotional strain on the care givers themselves which is often overlooked in research owing to a focus upon the patient's well-being. The range of research interests within the broad field of psychiatric oncology covers a plethora of psychosocial aspects of cancer from the initial assessment and diagnosis through to the issues of survivorship

(Chaturvedi et al 2003). Whereas the medical side of oncology focuses upon the biochemical features of carcinoma, psychiatric oncology focuses its attention upon a holistic approach to the emotional and behavioral care of the patient and of the support network surrounding the patient. Not just the emotional response to the diagnosis but to the on-going nurture of the patient's sense of self and well-being constitutes a major component of psychiatric oncology including the care and nurture of the care givers themselves in dealing with terminal cancer patients.

Although controversy and debate over the years has characterized research on the role of stress in the life of a cancer patient running the full gamut from diagnosis, prognosis, and survival, there is general clinical consensus that the recurrence of cancer often follows bereavement and the onset of a malignancy. Clearly the most common response of a patient diagnosed with cancer is fundamentally psychological and emotional in which life-threatening anxiety and fear of death are present. Accompanying the emotional and behavioral manifestations of stress and anxiety are the inevitable physical symptoms such as pain, nausea, as well as the anticipated effects of the medical, surgical, and radiation treatments with special concerns for the side effects of chemotherapy. Chaturvedi and colleagues (1996) are also quick to call attention to what has become decreasingly relevant in cancer care and that is the long-standing stigma characterizing a patient with cancer, more common in India and developing countries but still present somewhat in the West. Though western responses to cancer diagnosis vary somewhat but not profoundly from that of the Indian patient, the most commonly shared coping mechanisms employed by the patient include a blanket denial of the diagnosis, a turning to religious attachments, and inevitably the sense of outright helplessness and even hopelessness.

Studies conducted by Chaturvedi and his research colleagues all affirm the common presence of the psychiatric disorder of debilitatingly acute depression and anxiety but their clinical investigations have shown that there is a tendency to down-play the psychological morbidity among cancer patients themselves such that data on the prevalence and intensity of depression and anxiety are necessarily flawed. A wide swatch of clinical studies have shown that there is a prevalence of psychiatric morbidity among cancer patients (Chaturvedi et al, 1994), particularly that of depression, delirium, and anxiety disorders but much less frequently that of personality disorders, psychoses, and substance abuse. Chaturvedi and team found between 38% and 53% of cancer patients had identifiable psychiatric disorders using the *Diagnostic and Statistical Manual of*

Mental Disorders-III-R guide for identification. They found that in hospice-sponsored programs, general hospitals, and neurosurgery departments, psychiatric disorders were present at a 48% rate of which most were adjustment disorders. However, in cases where the cancer patient was resident in a cancer-based hospital, upwards of 53% manifested psychiatric disorders broken down into 22% depression, 15% sleep disorders, and 9% adjustment disorders. The most frequently evidenced psychiatric disorder across all clinical studies (Derogatis et al 1983) conducted early in the 1980s showed depression as the most common syndrome with 68% of all cancer patients manifesting these symptoms.

For decades, cancer treatment centers throughout the world have recognized that of those behavioral responses which are most prevalent and debilitating to the patient are depression and anxiety. Such depressive symptoms may result from the encroachment of the disease in course of development or as a response to the chemotherapeutics employed in the cancer treatment itself. Ironically yet understandably, the treatment modality may be as contributory to the rise of depression in the patient as knowledge of the cancer itself for depression commonly appears as a direct functional response to the initial cancer diagnosis and subsequent treatment. Psychiatric oncologists have found that both deep feelings of worthlessness as well as acute feelings of guilt on the part of the patient often serve as a discriminating differential between what would be considered from a psychiatric perspective as a normal and understandable sense of sadness and that of an incapacitating cancer-driven depression. Chaturvedi and colleagues have found in their clinical studies that the presence and persistence of a conspicuous level of debilitating depression varies considerably ranging from less than 2% to as high as 50% within diagnosed patients with a mean average of 24%. Other factors contributing to this range of depression include such things as the cancer site itself, the clinical course of advancement and type of treatment, and always the presence of pain within the patient is a key factor, with such prevalence of major depression ranging upwards of 40%.

Medical oncology researchers as well as psychiatric oncologists are fully cognizant of the range of problems resulting from a diagnosis of cancer which leads to clinical depression. The monumental challenge facing the diagnostician is attempting to determine whether the presenting symptoms of depression are directly linked to the cancer itself or the result of the psychological response to the announcement of the diagnosis to the patient's self-image and sense of well-being. Clinical research has shown, for instance, that symptoms frequently characterizing malignancy include such somatic factors as loss of appetite, loss of weight, insomnia, loss of concentration, and a loss of energy. Identifying organic somatic symptoms poses a particular challenge to the clinicians which has led to a shifting of focus away from somatic and towards psychological symptomatology thus differentiating symptoms linked to the disease itself and those linked to the psychosocial factors more readily subject to a psychiatric oncological assessment (Holland, 1986; Endicott 1984; Rapp 1989; Chaturvedi, 1990). Exacerbating the diagnostic attempts by the oncology team in determining the etiology and precipitant causes of depression in the cancer patient include a range of disparate factors such as the patient's age and gender, various palliative treatments, severe and unremitting pain but also such things as social isolation felt by the diagnosed patient, socioeconomic pressures and anxieties, mood disorders and substance abuse.

Though psychiatric oncologists have been engaged in on-going research of cancer patient behavioral patterns for decades, there has still to be the development of a one-size-fits-all patient profile and there probably never will be since psychosocial and cross-cultural factors loom large in the variable package involved in such research. Zigmond and Snath (1983) have shown that the Hospital Anxiety and Depression Scale (HADS) employed in India among cancer patients in major medical facilities have proven of some help in the categorization of depression and anxiety severity though Chaturvedi and team (1990, 1991) have consistently shown the short-comings in this profiling mechanism across a range of Asian populations. On the other hand, there has been some evidential success in measurement according Chaturvedi (1991, 1994) when using the Coping and Concerns Checklist (CCC). This measurement instrument was developed in India at the Cancer Research Campaign's Cancer Research Centre for it is somewhat helpful in the detection of both common physical as well as psychosocial problems in cancer patients. One interesting and surprising finding is that in the area of personal relationships only infrequently were such concerns as partnership relations, support from one's family, and sexual behavior. In these studies there was good reason to notice, according to the research team, that there was a diminishment of reported concern in these areas by the patient owing to the cultural censorship of complaints dealing with such relationships. Such cultural censorship inevitably diminished the significance of these findings.

Psychiatric oncologists have made a point of clinically differentiating between anxiety and depression. Anxiety is usually related to the normal stress of a reported cancer diagnosis leading commonly to adjustment disorders and delirium. Depression, on the other hand, is much more common among cancer patients than is generalized anxiety for only in carefully monitored clinical studies does the frequent lumping of anxiety and depression symptomatology occurs. Anxiety resulting from a cancer diagnosis is usually manifested in symptoms of persistent tension and worry, panic attacks, and palpitations resulting from concerns about the future, one's family finances, fear of relapses and recurrences once treatment has been completed and the enduring concern over survival issues affecting the family. These commonly present worries have easily been identified through the use of the Coping and Concerns Checklist (CCC). Thanks to advanced research by psychiatrists dealing with post-war traumas, psychiatric oncologists have been able to focus their attention upon the surprising presence of post-traumatic stress disorders (PTSD) not unlike war veterans. Recent CCC researchers have shown that cancer patients encounter such debilitating stress when abnormal growth is detected in their diagnosed cancer as well as the experience of hospitalization and treatment protocols such as radiation and chemotherapy. Researchers have noticed that somatoform symptoms often actually occur in recovering patients from cancer treatment in the form of fatigue, tiredness, and even pain which are assessed by the psychiatric oncologists as "abnormal illness behavior" (AIB). These manifestations are commonly misunderstood as a recurrence or relapse of the carcinoma leading to clinical management problems often resulting in either delayed or cancelled treatment (Chaturvedi et al 1993; Chaturvedi, Maguire 1998).

The rise of psychiatric oncology and the elevated position of the treatment team has been greatly enhanced by the effectiveness of the diagnostic recognition that the identification of cancer in a patient constitutes the greatest emotional reaction of any other disease related to mortality. Clinical studies show that "shock and disbelief" constitute the most common immediate reaction of the patient (and supporting family) with the subsequent emergence of anger, depression, and a sense of both loss and grief. The overall intensity and duration of these emotional responses vary with the individual and the psychiatric oncology team is trained to identify those characteristics and to respond accordingly. A plethora of behavioral and emotional responses on the part of the patient commonly following the diagnosis include such feelings as denial, anxiety, depression and even guilt. In India as in the U.S. often patients resort to their religious orientations for consolation (even drawing from childhood understandings of their faith). The most common overall fear on the part of the patient and the patient's family is that of the incurability of the disease and the inevitability of pain, discomfort, and helplessness in dealing with finality and issues of survivorship. Often, the stress and anxiety experienced by the family when confronted with a terminal diagnosis of its member is linked to financial concerns involving both the cost of treatment as well as the loss of income resulting from the anticipated death of the patient.

Clinical researches conducted by Chaturvedi (1996) and Chandra (et al., 1998) have shown that reactions to radiation treatment, while initially unpleasant with most uncomfortable side effects such as vomiting and severe fatigue, over time initial anxiety which at first was severe began to decline over time as treatment with radiotherapy continued and a subsequent adjustment and even acceptance of the treatment became somewhat normatively acceptable by the patient. Of the three common modalities of treatment – surgery, chemotherapy, radiation therapy – chemotherapy early on was considered least desirable owing to the frequency and intensity of nausea and vomiting but with the increasing sophistication of pharmacological interceptors, these side effects have greatly been reduced if not completely done away with. In cases where advanced cancer produced an increase in psychiatric morbidity, there are three fundamental reasons for this, viz., physical symptoms such as pain, nausea, vomiting and emotional distress, fear of death itself, and psychiatric disorders resulting from the metastasis of the cancer and its unstoppable progression (Chaturvedi, 1998).

Many psychiatric aspects of palliative care of the terminally diagnosed cancer patient besides detection and management of various emotional and behavioral issues is the challenge of meaningful communication with the patient and supportive family regarding survival issues. Over the years in the development of the specialization of psychiatric oncology, the medical team has found that the cultivation of skills in dealing with the issues of patient death anxiety often constitutes a more challenging agenda than dealing with the biophysical problems confronting the diagnosed patient. Chandra and research team (1999; 2008) have found that if the medical staff are taught to be more passive and responsively communicative rather than aggressively interventionistic both patients and family members are more likely to experience an easing of their anxiety and the diminishment of depression. A profoundly insightful database study conducted by Chochinov and colleagues (1995) addressing the issue of the patient's expressed desire for death found that both the prevalence and intensity of the desire to hasten death was directly related to such variables as demographics, psychiatric, psychosocial, and cancer variables. In their use of the Desire for Death Scale (DDS) in a clinical study of 191 cancer patients, there was actually no expressed desire for death among 34% of the patients with only 2% expressing an extreme desire which most commonly was present among widowed and divorced patients (Chaturvedi et al, 1994).

Over the years, more and more psychiatric oncologists have come to realize the central importance of cultivating communication skills regarding cancer diagnoses between the medical team (doctors and nurses) and the individual patient and family members. One danger which is always looming over the patient and family is the issue of collusion wherein the family is eager to collaborate with the medical team in "hiding" the bad news from the patient about the cancer diagnosis. Chaturvedi and Chandra (2010) have studied this challenge carefully and the data suggests that this tendency in the long run works to the disadvantage of all concerned. Chaturvedi and research colleagues (2008; 2010) are insistent upon the crying need for the medical staff to be specifically and intentionally trained in communicating bad news to patients and family members for up until most recently the medical staff has not been trained in such skills often to disastrous results in dealing with the cancer patient and the family. Too often, such communication failure leads to a decline in confidence in the quality and type of care being provided. In those reported cases where the medical team has been specifically trained in such sensitive communication skills using a workshop format, the effectiveness of the training has been linked to interactive discussions, role playing, video demonstrations and various teaching methods employed by professionals who have shown a particular skill in confronting these communication challenges.

In the last twenty years, the use of psychopharmacological intervention in the treatment of depression within the cancer patient has become increasingly common and reportedly effective, especially in the use of such medications as tricyclic antidepressants and specific serotonin reuptake inhibitors (SSRIs), monoamine oxidas inhibitors (MAOI), sympathomimetic stimulants, lithium carbonate, and less frequently alprazolam. Earlier studies suggested that the disinclination to employ antidepressants was the misplaced fear of addiction and the false assumption that the patient would eventually move beyond the need for such pharmaceutical assistance (Chaturvedi, Hopwell, Maguire, 1994; Chaturvedi, Chandra, 1996) but clinical studies have more recently and emphatically disproven the legitimacy of this fear.

The early recognition by Jimmie Holland, M.D. at the Sloan Kettering Cancer Center of the need for psychological management of the cancer patient led eventually to the development of the specialization in oncology of psychiatric oncology wherein the management of the patient's overall psychosocial well-being constitutes a fundamental agenda of the overall holistic medical care of the cancer patient. The legitimate recognition of the patient's expressions of anxieties, desires, hopes, and fears were embraced by the psychiatric oncologists as the right and proper focus of emotional health. The employment of psychotherapeutic modalities of treatment has become a standard operating practice within oncological care of the cancer patient such that individual and group counseling sessions, cognitive behavioral therapies, desensitization and rehabilitation mindfulness sessions have all become standard stock in trade in the care of patients. The not uncommon disinclination of the medical team, particularly the oncologists and physicians responsible for the primary care of the cancer patient, to make meaningful enquiries into the emotional well-being of the patient has proven to be a stumbling block in the effective long-term management of the psychological health of the cancer patient.

The challenge for well-trained oncologists and medical staff who are very good at the medical side of health care treatment is to understand that the cancer patient is otherwise a whole person suffering from severe stress and anxiety owing to the cancer diagnosis. Therefore, the patient stands in need of being treated as a whole person and not merely as a clinical case of terminal carcinoma! Those medical professionals involved as psychiatric oncologists in the comprehensive oversight of the whole patient are trained in three levels of sensitivity growing out of the counseling relationship with the terminal patient. First, there is the intake session in which the psychiatric oncologist is called upon with a high level of sensitivity on the part of the medical professional to glean as much personal information from the patient as possible involving physical conditions and symptoms, family histories, life experiences, etc. in an attempt to get a fuller picture of the patient's life prospects. Secondly, the opportunity is presented for the patient to be more fully forthcoming in terms of their own emotional state of mind and a sense of well-being or otherwise. Finally, this last level of counseling interaction is at the heart of the patient's willingness to be completely open about such feelings of death and survival issues such that the most practical questions regarding physical decline and death and post-death issues related to family concerns are able to be dealt with candidly, openly, and honestly.

One of the enduring questions, posed early in the development of psychiatric oncology, is whether or not that which is being gained by clinical researchers involved in the psychosocial care and treatment of cancer patients is actually of any real value to the patient in terms of the quality of life (QOL) issues or, are the findings more theoretically relevant to a deepening understanding of the complexities of carcinoma upon the human psyche as well as its somatic impact. The psychiatric oncology community is quick in their subsequent clinical studies to emphasize the evidentiary findings of the improvement or maintenance of a quality of life and well-being of the patient as the patient is led to a broader understanding of the cancer from which they are suffering and as a collaborative member of the treatment protocol rather than a mere bystander upon whom apparent experiments are being conducted and treatments administered. Detection of psychiatric morbidity, for example, is an area of significant advancement in the field and a deepening and broadening of the skills needed by the medical team to introduce bad new and to assist the patient in the processing of the end-of-life issues affecting the surviving family. The discoveries involved in the advancement of psychiatric morbidity have led to a more effective identification and treatment of psychiatric disorders evidenced in cancer patients. In addition to enhancing the family's involvement with a family member diagnosed with cancer when handling fundamentally practical issues such as finances, physical toxicities of the patient in response to the chemotherapies used, and the recognition and management of the psychosocial changes occurring in the patient through the assessment, diagnosis, and treatment phases of the illness, psychiatric oncology has greatly advanced in understanding of the stress and anxiety the actual day-to-day practice of oncology has upon the medical staff, nurses and doctors alike. This knowledge has led to an increased appreciation of the pressure under which the medical team works while assisting the patient and their families in likewise dealing with the disease. This knowledge has led to the development of effective coping mechanisms in managing stress among the health care team members. Quality of patient care has been shown to be directly correlated to the emotional health of the medical team itself.

The politics of medical practice is a huge area of concern and research in psychiatric oncology for this specialization finds itself right in the middle of that matrix of administration decisions affecting patients as well as institutional costs and staff time investments. The question, "Who is in charge?" always arises within the medical institutional setting. Owing to the fact that psychiatric oncology is fundamentally multidisciplinary, sorting out the diagnostic and treatment protocols between the biomedical character of the carcinoma and the psychosocial nature of the cancer patient's life situation, the question is always present in the larger more well-funded medical institutions as to the use of medical, surgical, radiation oncology along-side of the psychosocial issues handled by the psychiatric oncologists. All of these decisions are shadowed with the big question of financing this multidisciplinary treatment, i.e., "Who pays and how?" When so many high-level professions are involved in the treatment protocol – medical and psychiatric – there is always the danger that the patient and the family are overlooked in the professional struggles for oversight and accountability within the medical care team itself. Issues dealing particularly with the quality of life and patient well-being are often answered differently by the biomedical team and that of the psychosocial team.

Finally, and certainly not to be smoothed over, is the fact that the practice of psychiatric oncology is characterized by a mine-field of ethical questions which are not easily dealt with but require attention beginning with the simplest yet extremely emotionally fraught with controversy and emotional danger. That is to say, whether or not and when if ever the patient is actually told the full scope of the cancer diagnosis. The ethically challenging slippery slope involves the dangers of inadvertent collusion between the medical team and the patient's family, i.e., a conspiracy of silence, and the inevitability of the loss of trust within the family/medical matrix of information sharing. The most heart-wrenching challenge where national insurance does not cover the costs of care is that of the fundamental complex of medical treatment options based on ability to pay. (Chaturvedi 2008). Macleod (2007) has shown in his clinical studies that issues related to palliative medicine and end of life issues involving questions about termination of life constitute a major point of stress for the medical institution and its staff as well as the patient and the patient's family (Kandasamy et al 2011; Chaturvedi, Loiselle, Chandra 2009). The latest benefits realized by the on-going advancement of psychiatric oncology including the use of psychopharmacological intervention in cancer care (Grassi, Nanni, Uchitomi, Riba 2011) all conspire to validate the furtherance of this specialization in cancer patient care. The future is bright even within the context of challenges involving training and financing of this specialized field of oncology.

CHAPTER EIGHT
PSYCHIATRIC ONCOLOGY IN REVIEW

Two Decades and More of Pivotal Research

As has been discussed in detail earlier in these critical essays, the emergence of an awareness of and the need for research directed towards a deeper understanding of the emotional and behavioral issues confronting the cancer patient has been well documented. The formalized recognition within the medical establishment of psychiatric oncology has been slower in coming since the 1970s but today clearly this specialization has gained international acceptance. Medical institutions, both research and treatment oriented, have risen to the challenge of integrating an understanding of the psychosocial spectrum of issues affecting the quality of care and treatment of the cancer patient and family members involved such that today there is a full range of services at a large contingent of cancer centers and hospitals focusing both research and treatment upon the biomedical side as well as the psychosocial side of cancer diagnosis and protocols of care.

The scholarly journals early on responded to the realization that this specialization was here to stay and commenced publishing articles, both data-based and clinical, such that in the past five decades there have been hundreds of collaborative studies published in the international arena elevating the sophistication of psychiatric oncology to a high level of relevance. In the following, we have chosen a dozen articles published over the past twenty years which are indicative of the quality of work being done by medical academics and scholars. These articles are chosen because they are representative of the range and scope of scholarship in the field and are not promoted as the best of the best but as illustrative of the growing sophistication of research scholarship both in the U.S. and internationally. These selected articles have been treated chronologically and each treatment will begin with a simple bibliographic citation followed by a summary comment or two indicating their relevant place in the development of the specialization of psychiatric oncology.

Berard, R.M. (2001). "Depression and Anxiety in Oncology: The Psychiatrist's Perspective." *Journal of Clinical Psychiatry.* #62 Supplement 8:58-61; discussion 62-63.

Over twenty years ago, Berard called attention to the prevalence of both depression and anxiety in the lives of individuals diagnosed with cancer which commonly went unrecognized and seldom treated. He points out that the negative affect upon the cancer patient was sometimes frequently overlooked or discounted as an irrelevant factor in the treatment protocol. The result of this indifference resulted in a sparsity of clinical studies of this phenomenon even though there were at the time several pharmacotherapies employed in the treatment of depression and anxiety but not used in the treatment of cancer patients. Berard and clinical colleagues called attention to the Hospital Anxiety and Depression Scale (HADS) as one of an effective data-gathering tools addressing this void in current research and in this article he illustrates the effectiveness of diagnoses and treatment of both depression and anxiety in the improvement of the emotional well-being of cancer patients. He summarizes several treatment modalities employed at the time in oncological settings and shows how the HADS can effectively identify through screening various psychiatric and emotional issues experienced by the patient early in the diagnostic and treatment plan. At the time of writing, he reminds the reader that selective serotonin reuptake inhibitors are the most popular pharmacological treatments at the time which also clinically showed effectiveness in treating anxiety disorders as well. In this article, Berard and colleagues were calling for more pointed and aggressive clinical studies of the relationship between the biomedical and psychosocial care and treatment of the cancer patient.

Breitbart, W. S., Alici, Yesne (2009). "Psycho-Oncology." *Harvard Review of Psychiatry* #17(6): 361-376.

Nearly a decade after Berard's provocative article issuing the call for more research, Breitbart and Alici, writing for the *Harvard Review of Psychiatry,* drew specific attention to the clinical difficulties faced by oncology owing to the psychiatric sequelae of cancer which at the time was producing an increase in research and study addressing issues of screening, assessment, and management of these troublesome sequelae in the cancer patient. One overriding difficulty commonly confronting the treatment modalities employed at the time was the realization that various treatment protocols themselves can contribute to complications in the progression of the cancer being treated. As usually occurs, the development of a specialization within a technical field leads to the inevitable training programs for professionals seeking to focus attention upon the newly developing field and such has been the case with psychiatric oncology. About this time, medical centers specializing in cancer research and treatment commenced the aggressive training of social workers, psychologists, and general psychiatrists who chose to focus their practice specifically upon the behavioral and emotional care of the cancer patient and their families, ranging from initial diagnosis to survivorship.

Breitbart and Alici have offered in this essay a review of the general history of psycho-oncology including a listing of common psychological responses to cancer diagnosis on the part of both the individual and the family. Furthermore, they engaged in a brief but helpful overview of the assessment and management of various psychiatric illnesses and disorders commonly occurring in the cancer patient as well as offering a detailed discussion of the frequent occurrence of fatigue characterizing cancer treatment. Facilitating a deeper understanding of the central importance of the psychosocial character of cancer, Breitbart and Alici considered the various cognitive effects of cancer diagnosis and treatment protocols including the emotional care of the families leading up to and including bereavement and survivorship. Their general tone in this overview was to facilitate the effective sensitizing of the medical team designated to care for the patient and family through the entire process of early diagnosis, treatment, bereavement, and survivorship issues.

Sajatovic, M., Sanders, R., Alexeenko, L., Madhusoodanan, S. (2010). "Primary Prevention of Psychiatric Illness in Special Populations." *Annals of Clinical Psychiatry* Nov; 22(4): 262-273.

The year following the review essay of Breitbart and Alici saw an extremely helpful literature review done by Sajatovic, Sanders, Alexeenko, and Madhusoodanan which focused upon the fundamental prevention of psychiatric disorders in specifically identified populations such as those comprised of individuals who have at some juncture in life experienced a major emotional trauma, individuals in the military particularly with field experience, persons who have specific serious medical conditions prior to a cancer diagnosis, and more broadly based populations such as postpartum women and immigrants. The Sajatovic team was particularly focused upon populations who clinically showed a consistent susceptibility to psychiatric symptoms of mental disorders related to biographical episodes including both biological and socio-cultural features. Their review was particularly helpful in providing an overview of the range of medical literature addressing preventive issues in psychiatric symptomatology affecting both traumatized and abused victims, military personnel, cancer patients and patients with diabetes as well as pregnant and postpartum women and immigrants.

From the outset of their collaborative work in this review of literature, the Sajatovic team was fully cognizant of the glaring fact of the sparsity of published research on the fundamental issues dealing with the primary presence of mental illness in specialized populations such as has been listed above. Recognizing the practical realities of the general benefit of a universal prevention protocol promoted through public awareness, campaign awareness initiative, and disaster planning, it became clear to these researchers that a more specifically pointed and intensively directed interventionist agenda for special groups of individuals at greater risk of psychiatric disorders was unquestionably called for particularly in dealing with crisis counseling and severe traumatized individuals and groups. The consensus reached among the Sajatovic team of researchers was that a universal goal of primary prevention of mental illness might be effectively sought through specifically designed universally focused primary preventive measures addressing these particular specialized groups of susceptible individuals.

Sperner-Unterweger, B. (2011). “Psycho-oncology – Psychosocial oncology: Integration in a Concept of Oncological Treatment.” *Nervenarzt.* March; 82 (3): 371-378.

The German neurological journal, *Nervenarzt,* in the very next year in 2011 brought out an article by Sperner-Unterweger which highlighted a statistical reality generally understood within the medical establishment but which was relatively unknown within the general population, namely, that between 30 and 60% of cancer patients are frequently suffering from various other forms of psychosocial distress and psychiatric disorders. By defining psychiatric oncology as consisting of psychosocial aspects of prevention, etiology, diagnostics, treatment, rehabilitation, and survivorship, the parameters of this definition calls for an interdisciplinary approach to medical practice calling for an aggressive collaboration between the medical and the psychosocial professional staffing of the cancer care facilities. This study emphasized the importance of the recognition within the medical facility and attending professional staff that the overall aim of psychosocial care and treatment of the cancer patient is to establish and maintain a high level of quality of life for the patient and the family. Inevitably and necessarily this definitional collaboration calls for a conspicuously emphasized cooperation within the oncological team of psychiatrists and behavioral specialists. The overall protocol management of the care and treatment of the cancer patient, while falling generally to the primary oncologist in charge, necessarily requires a recognition of the specialized measures employed in the psychosocial and emotional care offered by particularly trained psychiatric and psychotherapeutic personnel within the treatment arena. Psychosocial intervention consists of the utilization of psychological and psychotherapeutic measures combined often with psychopharmacological components which are called for in the overall treatment protocol. The Sperner-Unterweger article was timely in emphasizing the crucial importance of collaboration within the overall medical team of care and treatment of the cancer patient involving both psychiatric and psychotherapeutic elements of care.

Haeck, M., Franke, S., Wiskemann, J., Mathiak, K. (2012). "Psycho-oncology." *Nervenarzt* Nov; 83(11)1468-1476.

Neurological studies related to cancer research have a strong record of insightful grasp of the holistic approach to patient care such that the relevance of the psychosocial aspects of oncological treatment has been given major consideration in the past two decades. The German periodical, *Nervenarzt* (Neurologist) has led the way in publishing significant studies related to psychiatric oncology and Haeck, Frane, Wiskemann, and Mathiak have been recognized leaders in this work. Their 2012 article on psychiatric oncology distinguished them as leaders in emphasizing the psychosocial care of cancer patients by demonstrating the central importance of the collaborative linking of biological, psychological, and social issues involved in the holistic care of the patient and the patient's family. They were among the first researchers to point out the fundamental relevance of what they chose to call "low-threshold" psychosocial support when fostering an interaction between cancer patient and relatives with the medical team of psychiatrists, oncologists, psychotherapists, and nursing staff. Haeck and team were among the first major researchers to call attention to the sparsity of interdisciplinary counseling and psychotherapy found in their clinical studies involving diagnostic and systematic screening of cancer patients. They emphasized the urgency for an acceleration of focused research involving a holistic approach to cancer patient care wherein there is fostered a balance between the biomedical and psychosocial attention to the overall well-being of the patient.

Mavrides, N., Pao, M. (2014). "Updates in Paediatric Psycho-Oncology." *International Review of Psychiatry* Feb; 26(1):63-73.

Less than a decade ago, a major essay was presented to the medical community by N. Mavrides and M. Pao published in the *International Review of Psychiatry* in which the state of pediatric and adolescent care of cancer patients at that time was elevated to the level of national recognition. Childhood oncology has a strong and vibrant history in the international medical community dating from the mid-1950s in the U.S. and England but Mavrides and Pao have illustrated that specialized attention to childhood cancer continues to need more focused research and treatment modalities. Realizing that 2% of all cancer patients in the U.S. involves children, i.e., between 12,000 and 14,000 children diagnosed with cancer each year, there has been a remarkable decline in morbidity owing to the aggressive and collaborative efforts of leading children's hospitals such as the Riley Children's Hospital and St. Jude's Children's Hospital, among others. In the last fifty years, they point out that the percentages have increased in survival rates from 10-20% for five year survivals early in the 20th century to better than 80% for five year survival rates in the early 21st century.

During this rapid acceleration of childhood survival, there has been a remarkable integration with childhood oncological practice of the recognition of the central importance of the psychosocial support of both children and parents. Incrementally slow but inevitably the psychiatric and oncological communities of medical practitioners have begun to embrace a holistic approach to the care of childhood cancer patients consisting of a positive balance of biomedical and psychosocial aspects of health and healing.

Begun initially as a referral protocol by oncologists directing patients and families to psychiatric and psychotherapeutic counseling services, there is now an aggressive integration of these two treatment modalities within the same cancer treatment institutions such that there is a clearly designed integrational collaboration amongst a medical team comprised of the attending nursing staff, psychiatry, psychotherapy, and oncology. Mavrides and Pao have focused this paper upon presenting to the medical community an updated package of psychosocial issues relevant to childhood medical practitioners dealing specifically with child cancer patients. They show how that pediatric psychiatric oncologists are faced with unique challenges in this specialization and have shown through a roster of researches listed in PubMed and PsychINFO databases that over the past decade from 2000 through 2013 a significant roster of relevant scholarship has been published using the key words of pediatrics, oncology, psychosocial care, family, siblings, cancer, psycho-oncology, psychosocial issues, depression, anxiety, survivorship, and end of life. This article constitutes a significant contribution to the dissemination of practical information in child psychiatric oncology.

Watson, Maggie, Dunn, Jeff, Holland, Jimmie C. (2014). "Review of the History and Development in the field of Psychosocial Oncology." *International Review of Psychiatry* Feb; 26 (1): 128-135.

As has been seen from the earlier discussion of the rise of this specialization, the name of Jimmie C. Holland, M.D., has played an important role in this development. In this 2014 article she is joined by Maggie Watson and Jeff Dunn in reviewing the historical development of what in the article is called "Psychosocial Oncology." Subsequently, Dr. Holland and colleagues at the Sloan Kettering Cancer Center altered the spelling of this specialization to that of "Psycho-Oncology," though her own professorship used the label "Psychiatric Oncology" (See Appendix C). Our assessment of this change in labeling has already been discussed in detail in Chapter Two above. This particular article is pivotal in establishing this specialization for in it the formal description is expounded and elaborated upon. Psychosocial oncology here is characterized as a "multi-disciplinary field of practice" for it portends to reach across medical, psychological, social, and behavioral aspects of the cancer patient's response to the diagnosis and treatment. Watson and colleagues explore generally the historical emergence of this new specialization in which there is the recognition of what is called a "changing ethos in medical practice" which allows for, even welcomes, this widening of oncology practice to include the emotional and behavioral side of the patient's diagnosis and treatment. Herein for the first time the use of the expression "modern psychosocial oncology" appears and is explained as covering a variety of relevant topics for research such as the diagnosis and handling of the psychological morbidity involved in a cancer diagnosis and resulting distress and anxiety which reaches across a full spectrum of emotional issues from the initial diagnosis to that of survivorship.

Owing to the breadth of this diagnostic spectrum, Watson and colleagues emphasize the need for the attending medical team to take full cognizance of the behavioral and lifestyle issues resulting in the life of both the patient and the family following the diagnosis such that inclusion of all relevant members – medical team, family, and patient – is essential in the development of a thorough-going treatment plan. These authors emphasize the relevance of "best practice" as endorsed by the international medical community's own established guidelines for assessment and treatment of cancer patients and these authorized practices are being increasingly and successfully combined to produce effective clinically verified results in patient care. In addition to such practices being briefly itemized and discussed in the essay, Watson, Dunn, and Holland make a strong case for the integration of the psychosocial and behavioral insights offered by both psychiatry and psychotherapy to be insinuated into the overall best practices mode of treatment. This article specifically mentions the crucial nature of a holistic approach to the care and treatment of the cancer patient facilitated by a medical treatment ethos of care which employs both the biomedical and psychosocial nature of cancer. This article proved profound in its impact.

Zielazny, P., Zielinska, P., de Walden-Galuszko, K., Kuziemski, K., Bethowska-Korpala, B. (2016). "Psychooncology in Poland." *Psychiatr. Pol.* Oct 31: 50(5): 1065-1073.

The significance of this article being included here rests upon the fact that it is a report from clinical researchers in Poland who have called attention to the work of their colleagues dating back to the late 1990s, recognizing that this specialization claims a history dating from the mid-1970s. Zielanzny and colleagues define psychiatric oncology by employing the definition of Watson, Dunn, and Holland (2014) in calling it an interdisciplinary field of medicine with an acknowledgement of the rightful place of the psychological features of cancer care and treatment of the diagnosed patient. They point out that psychiatric oncology is essentially a "sub-discipline of clinical oncology, psychiatry, clinical psychology and health psychology." Though leaving off psychotherapy as a major component of this collaborative enterprise, it is clear from the essay that psychotherapy and counseling psychology constitute a rightful component of the overall character of this sub-discipline. The historical relevance of this article is greatly enhanced by their referring to the establishment in Poland in 1992 of the Polish Psycho-Oncology Association created specifically to address this emerging specialization, acknowledging the central role played by Holland and company at the Sloan Kettering Cancer Center.

Though the Polish medical establishment recognized early on the great value gained from the emergence and employment of psychiatric oncology, these researchers are quick to point out that the national health insurance of Poland is insufficient in its recognition and coverage of this modality of treatment of Polish citizens diagnosed with cancer. The looming impediment to the further development of psychiatric oncology in the Polish medical system is the failure at the time of writing of defining psychiatric oncology and its practice by medical professionals such as to make it essentially an administratively separate and recognized professional specialization. Furthermore, there is the pressing need for the national insurance agencies in Poland to recognize and acknowledge the clinically verified efficacy of psycho-oncological benefits to the cancer patient by expanding the national health insurance plan to cover this treatment in the National Program of Cancer Prevention. This article was one of the first professional forays to present a formalized pivotal entrée into an international conversation regarding the benefits and efficacy of psychiatric oncology.

Kao, Larkin Elderon, Lokko, Hermioni N., Gallivan, Kathleen, O'Brien, Vera, Peteet, John R. (2017). "A Model of Collaborative Spiritual and Psychiatric Care on Oncology Patients." *Psychosomatics* Nov-Dec; 58 (6): 614-623.

In fairness to this article and in full disclosure of my own secular orientation, I have written in Appendix A an article titled "Religious Faith and Scientific Accountability: Exploring the False Conundrum in Medical Oncology." My article is extremely critical of attempts to integrate a "faith-based" perspective with a "science-based" perspective such that any indication of belief in divine intervention is out of place in a scientifically-oriented medical protocol. A colleague of mine, Prof. E. O. Wilson of Harvard, once said to me privately that the issue facing the religious and scientific communities is the realization that there is not and never can be a "faith-based science."

Kao and colleagues have emphasized in their opening comment in this article that they are venturing into unchartered waters when it comes to attempting to conjoin a treatment protocol consisting of chaplains (implying a "religious orientation") and consultation-liaison (C-L as it is labeled) psychiatrists (suggesting a "scientific orientation") during hospitalization treatment of cancer patients. They contend that various studies have indicated some sort of "healthy influence" between spirituality and mental health in which patients seem interested in their psychiatric team having some understanding of the patient's sense of spirituality or religious orientation. Kao and colleagues do admit early in the essay that there is currently (as of 2017) no published literature reflecting a clinical verification that patients prefer or desire or are even particularly receptive to a chaplaincy-psychiatry collaboration. This is a surmise on the part of the research team for this article is clearly and openly stated as in search for a positive interventionist model of bringing chaplains and psychiatrists together in a positive collaboration.

The venue in which the following extremely limited data-based clinical study was conducted was at the Brigham and Women's Hospital which is the second largest teaching hospital of Harvard Medical School and the largest hospital in the Longwood Medical Area in Boston, Massachusetts. Conducted over a nine month period in 2015 by the Consultation-Liaison Services at the hospital, the study consisted of 13 sessions drawing from chaplains and psychiatrists engaged in an interdisciplinary roundtable discussion of issues commonly confronted in the care of cancer patients. Eighteen individual patients participated by completing a questionnaire including both quantitative and qualitative prompts covering the before and after sessions ending with a study of the conclusions.

Admittedly an extremely limited data-base study where eighteen cancer patients actually completed the baseline questionnaire, upwards of 36% of the participants, i.e., 6 patients, described their experience as "very satisfied" whereas those "not comfortable" dealing with faith-based issues declined to 17% i.e., 3 patients. To questions seeking attitudes regarding how these discussions had been helpful to the patient the response was 83%, i.e., 15 patients, with reportedly all participants preferring an interdisciplinary approach. Kao and team continued to emphasize that to their own knowledge there had not been at the time of their study any other attempts based on clinical findings that sought the creation of a model drawing upon a collaborative participation between chaplaincy and Consultative-Liaison psychiatry. Never once was the issue of faith vis-à-vis science mentioned nor how faith-based clergy and science-based medical professionals could deal with this disparity of divine versus biochemical intervention in patient care.

Patel, S.B., McCall, W.V. (2020). "Interface of Psychiatric Services with Urological Oncology Practice." *European Urology Focus*. 05 May, 6(6):1140-1141.

In a very cryptic and succinct affirmation of the potentially positive relationship between the biomedical and psychosocial psychiatric approach to the care of the cancer patient, Patel and McCall have distinguished themselves in identifying clearly the benefits of developing a treatment modality designed to elevate an awareness of the patient's illness from a confluence of perspectives. They call for psychiatric participation in the overall cancer care team for it allows for a holistic assessment and treatment plan. By drawing from emotional, behavioral, and cognitive components of the patient's lifestyle, there is an attempt to reduce various social and even occupational impairments which eventuate in the treatment plan. This move is designed to improve the quality of life of the patient while monitoring the effectiveness of the overall treatment plan which involves both the biomedical as well as the psychosocial components of care.

Quante, Aim, Schulz, Kristina, Fissler, Maria (2020). "Psychiatric Comorbidities in Cancer Patients: Acute Interventions by the Psychiatric Consultation Liaison Service." *Wiener Medizinische Worchenschrift* Oct; 170 (13-14): 348-356.

Quante, Schulz, and Fissler provided an extremely valuable service in this data-base study for though much research had been done during the first two decades of the 21st century, there was a genuine sparsity of enquiries into the relationship between cancer and mental health and the interrelationship of a cancer diagnosis and the impact which results in the emotional well-being of the patient. Quante and colleagues addressed just this issue by calling attention to the importance of exploring the psychiatric comorbidities of individual cancer patients who had been examined by what was becoming a common classification of services called Consultation Liaison Psychiatry (CLP) appearing increasingly in general service hospitals (in this case Germany but commonly in England as well). Their intent was to provide an overview of the various psychiatric treatment modalities which were recommended most frequently by the CLP when addressing the connection between specifically identified cancer types and designated psychiatric disorders.

Over a one year period, the research team studied some 119 psychiatric cases in which consultations with cancer patients covered a full range of demographic details, cancer diagnostic statistics, psychiatric diagnoses and subsequent procedural treatment modalities. In this study group of patients, one third of the patients were treated either for hematological cancer or secondarily for lung cancer. The remaining two thirds covered a full spectrum of cancer types. The research team found that depression was the most common psychiatric disorder among all members of the study group. As detailed in this study, depression was certainly the most common emotional disorder found among cancer patients, up to one third of all cancer patients, and one third of all patients suffering from hematological cancer were diagnosed with both depression and delirium.

This study shows that the CLP recommended psychiatric treatment, when accompanied with psychotherapy (being the most common modality of treatment by the consulting psychiatric team) found that over 80% of all cancer patients studied received antidepressant medication based on the CLP recommendations along with psychotherapy. Quante and colleagues concluded that the data produced by the CLP demonstrated the central importance of early detection and initiating early treatment modalities appropriate to the cancer diagnosis owing to the presence of commonly existing comorbid psychiatric disorders which commonly accompany cancer patients.

Westermair, A.L., Schreiber, W., Dumchen, J., Perrar, K. M. (2020). "Psychiatrists in Palliative Care of People with Severe Psychiatric Illnesses and an Oncological Comorbidity." *Nervenarzt* May; 91 (5): 404-410.

Westermair, Schreiber, Dumchen, and Perrar have offered a very helpful essay on a topic which should occupy every major research institution dealing with the palliative care of the cancer patient with comorbidity issues. In their study they emphasize how demanding and challenging within the medical community is the treatment of oncology patients who are concurrently suffering from psychiatric disorders while being cared for within a medical palliative care institutional setting. To oncology specialists, the complicating features of psychiatric distress are commonly perceived as nearly overwhelming if not incomprehensible. To the cancer patient the experience of acute depression and debilitating delusional behavior within the overall context of a chronic psychotic attack can be severely frightening to both the patient and decidedly disturbing to the medical team attending the patient. Westermair and colleagues attempt in this essay to draw up an outline of epidemiological data which includes the various episodes experienced by this particular patient population. The overall insights which grew out of this study are presented as illustrative of case studies from a psychological perspective including psychiatric and palliative care issues all within the context of what has become commonly classified as psychiatric oncology.

Michaud, L., Stiefel, F. (2022). "Psychiatric Liaison II: Training." *Revue Medicale Suisse* 01 Feb, 18(769)265-268.

Most recently the French medical journal *Revue Medicale Suisse* published an article by Michaud and Stiefel continuing a discussion of the contributions being made by liaison psychiatry over the past two decades. In this essay they call attention to the communication skills which are involved in the training of oncologists with special emphasis upon the developing arena of behavioral and emotional components of cancer patient care. The gradual but inevitable inclusion of interpersonal dimensions of medical care of the cancer patient has elevated the quality of oncological treatment substantially by not only focusing upon the emotional well-being of the patient but of the medical staff's own personal self-understanding of their own worldview and ethos in treating terminally ill cancer patients. Michaud and Stiefel venture into a yet substantially unchartered territory of clinician-centered supervision training designed to raise to consciousness the psychological issues operative within the attending clinicians themselves. The intent is to bring to greater awareness the central importance of an understanding by the clinician of his or her own self-understanding of the nature of medical care within the context of a cognizance of their own operational worldview and ethos of care and treatment of the terminal patient. This recent article is considered a pivotal advancement in the field.

APPENDIX A
RELIGIOUS FAITH AND SCIENTIFIC ACCOUNTABILITY

Exploring the False Conundrum in Medical Oncology*

When religious answers fail the questioning cancer patient (and the family), the burden for answers shifts to science and the medical accountability for the inevitabilities of a terminal diagnosis. Dealing with the loss of faith or confidence in one's own religious orientation (whether patient, family, or medical staff) constitutes a monumental and strategic challenge to the psychosocial care of the terminal patient. For the scientifically skilled medical team unwisely inclined to employ a contrived placebo of religious metaphor in a misguided effort to ease the struggles of a religiously oriented cancer patient constitutes both a medical ethics issue of major proportions and a best practices conundrum for the medical team. Whether or not a secular definition of religion would be acceptable within a medically trained community of scientifically oriented professionals who themselves are self-described as religious is quite a question to ponder elsewhere. In these acute situations religion often functions merely as a placebo for a desperately sought after idea of a compassionate God. When, however, religious metaphor fails to comfort, then it must be replaced by a rational acceptance of the inevitabilities of life thereby negating the role and legitimacy of the "religious counselor." This shift from metaphor to science permits an emphasis upon the immediacy of the meaning and value of life-in-the-moment as a procedural mode of emotional care. If, however, a religiously functioning placebo is thought by the attending medical team to be more immediately efficacious, even though understood by the team to be a placebo, then the procedural modality of terminal palliative care rests on the sense of fair play in the minds of the attending medical team. The ethics of such a decision is quite profoundly substantial.

There are several typologies relevant in the study of the relationship between the presence of religion in the terminal oncology patient and sound medical practice. Four types are most commonly encountered within a care and treatment institution, viz., (a) the true believer who holds on to faith until the very end of life without hesitation or doubt (most frequently supported by a family and social matrix of likeminded individuals), (b) the patient whose confidence in a life of faith begins to falter over time and is eventually replaced by a nagging and unrelenting doubt, (c) the patient who at the beginning of the cancer is devoid or completely indifferent to the need of religious awareness but gradually and eventually reaches a point of sincere and persistent quest for a sustaining faith of whatever sort but always informed by a belief in life after death, and (d) that individual who intellectually and emotionally has chosen not to embrace any since of a transcendent reality which implies or requires a transcendent being.

All four types of patients are commonly found in patient treatment records of oncology clinics and hospitals with data-base statistics suggesting that in the United States upwards of half of the terminally ill cancer patient fall within type (a) with a gradual declining percentage falling into types (b) and (c) with only a small minority assuming that of type (d). In the following we take full cognizance of the fact that within the practice of oncology there is an extremely high percentage of health care providers who themselves are aligned with a religious faith, whether consciously articulated or subliminally embraced. The exacerbating circumstances in the treatment of the cancer patient in both types (b) and (d) when most often under the care of a medical team most commonly characterized by type (a) are evident throughout the literature which has explored the relationship between religious faith and medical accountability. One glaring methodological problematic suggestive of Heisenberg's "uncertainty principle" is that the researchers publishing their findings consistently fail to identify themselves within the typologies laid out in this discussion such that one is uncertain as to the ideological orientation towards religion of the researchers propounding a scientific exploration involving the relationship between religion and science. The abiding question must inevitably and forever be, is there any viability of seeking a convergence of a human construct (religion) and a scientific factuality (medicine)? Not being able to validate the claims of a religious belief in "life after death" as compared to the sheer reality of the physical death of the patient constitutes a monumental problem for medical practitioners.

We have chosen to refer to this matrix of embarrassingly overlooked or ignored field of research involving both the patient, whose faith recedes during the course of the illness (type b), and that patient who has no emotional attachment to the concept of faith at all (type d) as the "last taboo" within oncological medical practice. The problematics of raising the topic within scholarly discourse of the last taboo has to-date been more or less banished from polite medical investigations. Anyone in the profession who ventures into tabooed territory suffers the prospects of professional isolation. The last taboo prevents the medical team from candor regarding their own religious orientation and prevents the medical team from venturing into the troubling waters of separating their own faith from science and their own medical practice. Therefore, the patient without a religious orientation as well as the patient who begins with faith and ends with doubt is left moribund and isolated from what should be the purview of the emotional care of the patient provided ostensibly by psychiatric oncology. This clearly is a false conundrum created by a failure of the medical team to come to a self-reflective consciousness of their own orientation towards the necessity of a differentiation between personal faith and professional science and an established protocol related to the care of patients falling within all four typologies.

*This Special Report is taken from the *Quarterly Review of Clinical Psychopathology I.IV.2022*

Special thanks for postdoctoral appointments to the Divinity Schools of Harvard, Yale, Princeton, the University of Chicago and as the National Science Foundation Science Faculty Fellow at the University of Notre Dame wherein these thoughts first germinated.

APPENDIX B
MEDICATION AND COUNSELING IN PSYCHIATRIC PRACTICE:
Biogenic Psychopharmacology and Psychogenic Psychotherapy

(Partnering in the Treatment of Mental Illness)

The practice of psychiatry, though a very young specialization within the field of medicine, was historically restricted to practitioners holding the Doctor of Medicine degree. It covered a wide ranging field of interests and clinical practices, including but not restricted to a combination of psychotropic drugs and psychotherapy. Since the coming of Harry Stack Sullivan (1892-1949), psychiatry has been redefined by him and his colleagues at the William Alanson White Institute of Psychiatry in New York City and the Washington School of Psychiatry in D.C. as "the study of processes that involve or go on between people. The field of psychiatry," then, he suggested, "is the field of interpersonal relations, under any and all circumstances in which these relations exist." Not everyone in or out of medical practice agree with Sullivan and his colleagues but the sentiment within the broader counseling profession is that this more expansive and psychogenic definition is now more commonly employed in today's complex world of clinical psychotherapeutic and medical practice than is the old traditional and restricted biogenic definition circumscribed by psychotropic medical intervention.

Medication and counseling, and a varying combination of the two, constitute what today is thought of as the appropriate treatment for mental disorders. Based on whether the diagnosis of the presenting mental disorder is biogenic or psychogenic in nature, either psychotropic drugs or psychotherapy must necessarily dictate the treatment prescribed. Psychopharmacology and psychotherapy are both considered appropriate methods of treatment depending, of course, on the diagnosis. The present state of psychiatry, dominated by the insurance industry's jurisdiction in terms of coverable fee-based treatment, has been somewhat restricted in the use of psychotherapy in deference to psychopharmacological intervention. Within and without the profession there is the general consensus that the practice of psychiatry has suffered from these fiscal constraints and, therefore, a reliance upon social workers trained in counseling has become the normative practice within psychiatric treatment when a psychogenic illness has been diagnosed.

If Sullivan and company's expanded definition of psychiatry is embraced, namely, that this field of medicine deals fundamentally with interpersonal relationships, and the medical community is in agreement that both drugs and counseling are appropriate modalities of treatment, based upon the diagnosis, then a companioning of psychopharmacology and psychotherapy in psychiatric practice seems most reasonable and desirable. Biogenic illnesses are subject to psychopharmacological treatment whereas psychogenic illnesses are the domain of psychotherapy. In the best of all possible worlds, a complimentary relationship of these two modalities of treatment constitutes the ideal situation in any clinical practice. One need not adhere to the extremism of Thomas Szasz to see the value in pursuing a balanced diagnosis and treatment of mental illness using both drugs and counseling. The exploration of both modalities of treatment, pointing out the value of each within their own perimeters of jurisdiction and practice, would constitute a significant contribution to the discussion of the relationship between medication and counseling in the treatment of mental illness and the nurturing of mental health.

APPENDIX C

JIMMIE C. HOLLAND, M.D. (1928 – 2017)

No one questions the fact that Jimmie Coker Holland (April 9, 1928 – December 24, 2017) is the creator of the field of psychiatric oncology which came about during her years of service in psychiatric care at the Memorial Sloan Kettering Cancer Center in New York where she and colleagues taught psychologists how to deal with the psychosocial issues confronting cancer patients. After earning her medical degree in 1952 at the Baylor College of Medicine in Houston, Texas, she sought board certification in psychiatry and subsequently taught and practiced at the Montefiore Hospital of Albert Einstein College of Medicine in New York. From 1977 to 1996, she held the Wayne E. Chapman Chair in Psychiatric Oncology and was chief of Psychiatric Services at the Memorial Sloan-Kettering Cancer Center in New York where she developed a formal training program for teaching and research in psycho-oncology. She eventually founded the American Psychosocial Oncology Society in 1980 while editing the journal *Psycho-Oncology*. In 1994 she received the American Cancer Society's Medal of Honor for clinical research. She died in 2017 at the age of 89 from complications of cardiovascular disease.

BIBLIOGRAPHICAL REFERENCES AND RESOURCES

(Note: Though our focus has been upon published studies primarily during the past four decades, I have taken the liberty of listing some of the more profoundly important studies conducted by Asian scholars back to the 1980s.)

Abraham, Francis and John H. Morgan (1989). *Sociological Thought from Comte To Sorokin* (Levering, MI: Wyndham Hall Press).

Allexander, Frank G. and Sheldon T. Selesnick. *The History of Psychiatry: An Evaluation of the Psychiatric Thought and Practice from Prehistoric Times to the Present* (N.Y.: Jason Aronson, 1977).

Adams, Henry E. and Patricia B. Sutker (Editors). *Comprehensive Handbook of Psychopathology (3rd Edition).* (New York: Springer Publishing, 2004).

Adler, Alfred (1927). *Understanding Human Nature* (Garden City, NY: Garden City Publ.)

Antoni MH, Lutgendorf SK, Cole SW, Dhabhar FS, Sephton SE, McDonald PG, Stefanek M, Sood AK (March 2006). "The influence of bio-behavioural factors on tumour biology: pathways and mechanisms". *Nature Reviews. Cancer.* 6 (3): 240–8.

Balboni, M.J., Babar, A., Dillinger, J., Phelps, A.C., George, E., Block, S.D., Kachnic, L., Hunt, J., Peteet, J., Prigerson, H.G., VanderWeele, T.J., and Balboni, T.A. (2011). "It depends": "Viewpoints of patients, physicians and nurses on patient-practitioner prayer in the setting of advanced cancer. *Journal of Pain and Symptom Management*, 41:836-847.

Balboni, T.A., Balboni, M.J., Phelps, A.C., Wright, A.A., Peteet, J.R., Block, S.D., Lathan, C. VanderWeele, T.J., and Prigerson, H.G. (2011). "Support of terminal cancer patient spiritual needs and associations with medical care costs at the end of life." *Cancer*, 117:5383-5391

Balboni, T.A., Balboni, M.J., Enzinger, A.C., Gallivan, K., Paulk, M.E.,Wright, A., Steinhauser, K.,VanderWeele, T.J., and Prigerson, H.G. (2013). "Provision of spiritual support to advanced cancer patients by religious communities and associations with medical care at the end of life." *JAMA Internal Medicine*, 73:1109-1117.

Balboni, M.J., Sullivan, A., Amobi, A., Phelps, A.C., Gorman, D., Zollfrank, A., Peteet, J.R., Prigerson, H.G., VanderWeele, T.J. and Balboni, T.A. (2013). "Why is spiritual care infrequent at the end of life? Spiritual care perceptions among patients, nurses, and physicians and the role of training." *Journal of Clinical Oncology*, 30:2538-2544.

Balboni, M.J., Sullivan, A., Enzinger, A.C., Epstein-Petersen, Z., Tseng, Y., Mitchell, C., Niska, B.A., Zollfrank, A., VanderWeele, T.J., and Balboni, T. (2014). "Nurse and physician barriers to spiritual care provision at the end of life." *Journal of Pain and Symptom Management*, 48:400-410.

Balboni, M.J., Sullivan, A., Enzinger, A.C., Smith, P.T., Mitchell, C., Peteet, J.R., Tulsky, J., VanderWeele, T.J., and Balboni, T.A. (2017). United States clergy religious values and relationships to end-of-life discussions and care. *Journal of Pain and Symptom Management*, 53:999 Bower JE, Lamkin DM (March 2013). "Inflammation and cancer-related fatigue: mechanisms, contributing factors, and treatment implications". *Brain, Behavior, and Immunity.* 30 Supplement: S48–57.

Barskova T, Oesterreich R (2009). "Post-traumatic growth in people living with a serious medical condition and its relations to physical and mental health: a systematic review". *Disability and Rehabilitation.* 31 (21): 1709–33.

Berard, R.M. (2001). "Depression and Anxiety in Oncology: The Psychiatrist's Perspective." *Journal of Clinical Psychiatry.* #62 Supplement 8:58-61; discussion 62-63.

Berrios GE, Luque R, Villagran JM (2003). "Schizophrenia: a conceptual history" (PDF). *International Journal of Psychology and Psychological Therapy.* 3 (2): 111–140.

Bower, J. E., Lamkin, D. M. (2013). "Inflammation and Cancere-Relateed Fatigue: Mechanisms, contributing factors, and treatment implications." *Brain, Behavior, and Immunity.* 30 Supplement: S-48-57.

Breitbart, William; Rosenfeld, Barry; Gibson, Christopher; Pessin, Hayley; Poppito, Shannon; Nelson, Christian; Tomarken, Alexis; Timm, Anne Kosinski; Berg, Amy

(2016). "Meaning-centered group psychotherapy for patients with advanced cancer: a pilot randomized controlled trial". *Psycho-oncology*. 19 (1): 21–28.

Breitbart, W. S., Alici, Yesne (2009). "Psycho-Oncology." *Harvard Review of Psychiatry* #17(6): 361-376.

Breitbart, W. S. et al. *Psycho-Oncology* 4th Ed. (London: Oxford University Press, 2021).

Briole G (2012). *"Emil Kraepelin: The Fragility of a Colossal Oeuvre"*. Hurly-Burly. 8: 125–147.

Browne, Samuel and Meredith Burton. *The History of Psychiatry: Important Figures and Developments*. (Amazon, 2016).

Campbell, Robert Jean. *Campbell's Psychiatric Dictionary* (London: Oxford University Press, 2009, 9th Edition).

Carlson LE, Angen M, Cullum J, Goodey E, Koopmans J, Lamont L, MacRae JH, Martin M, Pelletier G, Robinson J, Simpson JS, Speca M, Tillotson L, Bultz BD (June 2004). "High levels of untreated distress and fatigue in cancer patients". *British Journal of Cancer*. 90 (12): 2297–304.

Carlson LE, Angen M, Cullum J, Goodey E, Koopmans J, Lamont L, MacRae JH, Martin M, Pelletier G, Robinson J, Simpson JS, Speca M, Tillotson L, Bultz BD (June 2004). "High levels of untreated distress and fatigue in cancer patients". *British Journal of Cancer.* 90 (12): 2297–304.

Chandra P, Chaturvedi SK, Channabasavanna SM, Anantha N, Reddy BK, Sharma S. "Subjective Well Being in Patients receiving Radiotherapy." *Qual Life Res.* 1998;7:495–500.

Chandra PS, Akhileswaran R, Chaturvedi SK, Shinde U. (1999). *Caring at home: frequently asked questions by persons with advanced cancers and their caregivers.* Bangalore: Published by BHT Center for Palliative Care Education.

Chapman, A. H. (1976). *Harry Stack Sullivan: History Life and His Work.* N.Y.P: G. P. Putnam's Sons.

Chaturvedi SK. "Asian Patients and the HAD Scales." *Br J Psychiatry.* 1990;156:133.

Chaturvedi SK. "Clinical irrelevance of HADS factor structure (for use in cancer patients)." *Br J Psychiatry.* 1991;159:298.

Chaturvedi SK. "Exploration of concerns and the role of psychosocial intervention in Palliative care." *Ann Acad Med Singapore.* 1994;23:756–60.

Chaturvedi SK. "Substituting nonsomatic for somatic symptoms in the diagnosis of depression." *Am J Psychiatry.* 1990;147:958–9.

Chaturvedi SK. "Exploration of concerns and the role of psychosocial intervention in Palliative care." *Ann Acad Med Singapore.* 1994;23:756–60.

Chaturvedi SK, Loiselle CG, Chandra PS. "Communication with relatives and collusion in palliative care – A cross cultural perspective." *Indian J Palliat Care.* 2009;15:2–9.

Chaturvedi SK, Chandra PS. "Breaking bad news- issues critical for psychiatrists. Medical Education corner." *Asian J Psychiatry.* 2010;3:87–89.

Chaturvedi SK. “Psychiatric Oncology.” In: Vyas JN, Nathawat SS, editors. *Psychiatry by Ten Teachers.* New Delhi: Aditya Medical Publishers; 2003. pp. 420–33.

Chaturvedi SK, Shenoy A, Prasad KMR, “Senthilnathan SM, Premkumari BS. Concerns, coping and Quality of life in head and neck cancers.” *Support Care Cancer.* 1996;4:186–90.

Chaturvedi SK, Chandra P, Channabasavanna SM, Pandian RD, Beena MB. “Detection of anxiety and depression in cancer patients.” *NIMHANS.* 1994;12:141–4.

Chaturvedi SK, Chandra PS, Channabasavanna SM, Anantha N, Reddy BK, Sharma S. “Levels of anxiety and depression in patients receiving radiotherapy in India.” *Psychooncology.* 1996;5:343–6. 22.

Chaturvedi SK, Loiselle CG, Chandra PS. “Communication with relatives and collusion in palliative care – A cross cultural perspective.” *Indian J Palliat Care.* 2009;15:2–9.

Chaturvedi SK, Chandra PS. "Breaking bad news- issues critical for psychiatrists. Medical Education corner." *Asian J Psychiatry.* 2010;3:87–89.

Chaturvedi SK, Chandra P. "Palliative Care in India." *Support Care Cancer.* 1998;6:81–4.

Chaturvedi SK. "Report of the Terry Fox Project on Quality of Life of cancer patients Bangalore." *NIMHANS*; 2003.

Chaturvedi SK, Hopwood P, Maguire GP. "Somatisation in cancer patients." *Eur J Cancer.* 1993;29A:1006–8.

Chaturvedi SK, Maguire P. "Persistent somatization in Cancer- a controlled follow-up study." *J Psychosom Res.* 1998;45:249–56.

Chaturvedi SK, Maguire P, Somashekhar BS. "Somatization in cancer." *Int Rev Psychiatry.* 2006;18:49–54.

Chaturvedi SK, Maguire P. "UICC World Congress Proceedings. Persistent fatigue in disease free cancer patients – a comparative study." *Medimond Publications*; 2006. pp. 271–420.

Chaturvedi SK, Venkateswaran C. "New Research in Psycho Oncology." *Curr Opin Psychiatry.* 2008;21:206–10.

Chochinov HM, Wilson KG, Enns M, Mowchun N, Lander S, Levitt M, et al. "Desire for death in the terminally ill." *Am J Psychiatry.* 1995;152:1185–91.

Consedine NS, Magai C, Krivoshekova YS, Ryzewicz L, Neugut AI (April 2004). "Fear, anxiety, worry, and breast cancer screening behavior: a critical review". *Cancer Epidemiology, Biomarkers & Prevention.* 13 (4): 501–10.

Cramer H, Lauche R, Paul A, Dobos G (October 2012). "Mindfulness-based stress reduction for breast cancer-a systematic review and meta-analysis". *Current Oncology.* 19 (5): e343-52.

Derogatis LR, Morrow GR, Fetting J, Penman D, Piasetsky S, Schmale AM, Henrichs M, Carnicke CL (February 1983). "The prevalence of psychiatric disorders among cancer patients". *JAMA.* 249 (6): 751–7.

Diagnostic and Statistical Manual of Mental Disorders (2013, 5th Edition). (Washington, DC: American Psychiatric Publishing.

DiMatteo MR, Lepper HS, Croghan TW. "Depression is a risk factor for noncompliance with medical treatment: meta-analysis of the effects of anxiety and depression on patient adherence". *Archives of Internal Medicine.* 2000: 160 (14): 2101–7.

Duffy James and Alan Valentine. (2011). *MD Anderson Manual of Psychosocial Oncology* (New York: McGraw Hill).

Ebert, Andreas. "Emil Kraepelin: A pioneer of Scientific Understanding of Psychiatry and Ppsychopharmacology". *US National Library of Medicine.* 2010: 52: 191–192.

Endicott J. "Measurement of depression in patients with cancer." *Cancer.* 1984;53:2243–7.

Engstrom EJ, Weber MM, Burgmair W. "Emil Wilhelm Magnus Georg Kraepelin (1856–1926)". The American Journal of Psychiatry. 2006: 163 (10): 1710.

Evans, F. B. (1996). *Harry Stack Sullivan: Interpersonal Theory and Psychotherapy.* N.Y.: Routledge.

Frankl, Viktor E. (1946). *The Doctor and the Soul: From Psychotherapy to Logotherapy* (N.Y: Bantam Books.

Freedheim, Donald K. (Editor). (1992). *History of Psychotherapy: A Century of Change* (Washington, DC: American Psychological Association).

Gabriel, Israel; Creedy, Debra; Coyne, Elisabeth (2020). "A systematic review of psychosocial interventions to improve quality of life of people with cancer and their family caregivers". *Nursing Open.* 7 (5): 1299–1312.

Gotay CC. "Behavior and cancer prevention". *Journal of Clinical Oncology.* 2005: 23 (2): 301–10.

Grassi L, Nanni MG, Uchitomi Y, Riba M. "Pharmacotherapy of depression in people with cancer." In: Kissane Maj M, Sartorius N, editors. *Depression and Cancer.* NY: John Wiley & Sons; 2011.

Greer JA, Park ER, Prigerson HG, Safren SA. "Tailoring Cognitive-Behavioral Therapy to Treat Anxiety Comorbid with Advanced Cancer". *Journal of Cognitive Psychotherapy. 20010:* 24 (4): 294–313.

Greer JA, Amoyal N, Nisotel L, Fishbein JN, MacDonald J, Stagl J, Lennes I, Temel JS, Safren SA, Pirl WF. "A Systematic Review of Adherence to Oral Antineoplastic Therapies". *The Oncologist.* 2016: 21 (3): 354–76.

Haeck, M., Franke, S., Wiskemann, J., Mathiak, K. "Psycho-oncology." *Nervenarzt 2012:*Nov; 83(11)1468-1476.

Hanahan D, Weinberg RA. "Hallmarks of cancer: the next generation". *Cell.* 2011 144 (5): 646–74.

Hoffman, Edward (1994). *The Drive for Self: Alfred Adler and the Founding of Individual Psychology* (New York: Addison-Wesley Publishing).

Hofmann SG, Sawyer AT, Witt AA, Oh D. "The effect of mindfulness-based therapy on anxiety and depression: A meta-analytic review". *Journal of Consulting and Clinical Psychology.* 2010: 78 (2): 169–83.

Holland JC. "Managing depression in the patient with cancer." *Clin Oncol.* 1986;1:11–3.

Holland, JC. *Handbook of Psychooncology: Psychological Care of the Patient with Cancer* (New York: Oxford University Press, 1989).

Holland, JC. "History of psycho-oncology: overcoming attitudinal and conceptual barriers". *Psychosom. Med.* 2002: 64 (2): 206–21.

Holland JC, Bultz BD. "The NCCN guideline for distress management: a case for making distress the sixth vital sign". *Journal of the National Comprehensive Cancer Network.* 2007: 5 (1): 3–7.

Holt-Lunstad J, Smith TB, Baker M, Harris T, Stephenson D. "Loneliness and social isolation as risk factors for mortality: a meta-analytic review". Perspectives on Psychological Science : *A Journal of the Association for Psychological Science.* 2015: 10 (2): 227–37.

Kandasamy A, Chaturvedi SK, Desai G. Spirituality, distress, depression, anxiety and quality of life in patients with advanced cancer. In*dian J Cancer.* 2011;48:55–9.

Kao, Larkin Elderon, Lokko, Hermioni N., Gallivan, Kathleen, O'Brien, Vera, Peteet, John R. "A Model of Collaborative Spiritual and Psychiatric Care on Oncology Patients." *Psychosomatics 2017:* Nov-Dec; 58 (6): 614-623.

Kraepelin, Emil (1906). *Über Sprachstörungen im Traume.* Leizpig: Engelmann.

Kraepelin, Emil (1987). *Memoirs.* Berlin, Heidelberg, New York: Springer-Verlag.

Kraepelin, Emil (2000). Vol. I: Persönliches, Selbstzeugnisse. Munich: Belleville.

Kraepelin, Emil (2001). Vol. II: Kriminologische und forensische Schriften: Werke und Briefe. Munich: Belleville.

Kraepelin, Emil (2002). Vol. III: Briefe I, 1868–1886. Munich: Belleville.

Kraepelin, Emil (2003). Vol. IV: Kraepelin in Dorpat, 1886–1891. Munich: Belleville.

Kraepelin, Emil (2005). Vol. V: Kraepelin in Heidelberg, 1891–1903. Munich: Belleville.

Kraepelin, Emil (2006). Vol. VI: Kraepelin in München I: 1903–1914. Munich: Belleville.

Kraepelin, Emil (2009). Vol. VII: Kraepelin in München II: 1914–1920. Munich: Belleville.

Kraepelin, Emil (2013). Vol. VIII: Kraepelin in München III: 1921–1926. Munich: Belleville.

Kröz M, Reif M, Büssing A, Zerm R, Feder G, Bockelbrink A, et al. "Does self-regulation and autonomic regulation have an influence on survival in breast and colon carcinoma patients? results of a prospective outcome study". *Health and Quality of Life Outcomes. 2011: 9*: 85.

Kwekkeboom KL, Cherwin CH, Lee JW, Wanta B. "Mind-body treatments for the pain-fatigue-sleep disturbance symptom cluster in persons with cancer". *Journal of Pain and Symptom Management.* 2010: 39 (1): 126–38.

Lee V. "The existential plight of cancer: meaning making as a concrete approach to the intangible search for meaning". *Supportive Care in Cancer*. 2008: 16 (7): 779–85.

Livesley, W. John and Roseann Larstone. (2018). *Handbook of Personality Disorders: Theory, Research, and Traetment* (New York: The Guilford Press).

Ludwig, Arnold M. (1980). *Principles of Clinical Psychiatry* (London: The Free Press).

Macleod AD. (2007). *The dying mind.* New York: Radcliff Publishing.

Maguire P, Heavens C. "Training hospice nurses in eliciting concerns." *Journal of Adv Nurs*. 1996;23:280–6.

Manis, Jerome G. and Bernard N. Meltzer (1972). *Symbolic Interaction: A Reader in Social Psychology,* 2nd Edition (Boston: Allyn and Bacon, Inc.)

Mavrides, N., Pao, M. "Updates in Paediatric Psycho-Oncology." *International Review of Psychiatry* Feb; 2014: 26(1):63-73.

Michaud, L., Stiefel, F. "Psychiatric Liaison II: Training." *Revue Medicale Suisse. 2022:* 01 Feb, 18(769)265-268.

Mitchell AJ, Chan M, Bhatti H, Halton M, Grassi L, Johansen C, et al. "Prevalence of depression, anxiety, and adjustment disorder in oncological, haematological, and palliative-care settings: A meta-analysis of 94 interview-based studies." *Lancet Oncol.* 2011;12:160–74.

Morgan, John H. (2015). *Clinical Psychotherapy: A History of Theory and Practice* (Lima, OH: Wyndham Hall Press).

Morgan, John H. (2018). *Harry Stack Sullivan: An Encyclopedic Dictionary of Interpersonal Psychotherapy* (Bristol, IN: MacBain & Boyd, Publishers).

Morgan, John H. (2021). *The Scope of Modern Psychiatry: Treatment Options in Clinical Practice.* (Lima,OH: Wyndham Hall Press).

Morgan, John H. (2021). *The Damaged Self: Exploring the Psychopathology of a Diminished Life* (Levering, MI: Wyndham Hall Press).

Morgan, John H. (2021). *A Summary Guide to the Collected Works of Sigmund Freud: The Freud Compendium* (Levering, MI: Wyndham Hall Press).

Morgan, John H. (2022). *Schizophrenia: The Enduring Challenge to Psychiatric Practice* (Levering, MI: Wyndham Hall Press).

Morgan, John H. (2019). *Child Psychopathology in Clinical Practice: The Psychoanalytic Theories of Karen Horney, Melanie Klein, and Anna Freud* (Levering, MI: Wyndham Hall Press).

Morgan, John H. (2020). *Psychopathology: A Clinical Guide to Personality Disorders* (Lima, OH: Wyndham Hall Press).

Morgan, John H. (2015; 2nd ed. 2017) *Clinical Psychotherapy: A History of Theory and Practice (from Sigmund Freud to Aaron Beck.* Mishawaka, IN: GTF Books.

Morgan, John H. (2017). *Understanding Ourselves: Essays in the History and Philosophy of the Social Sciences* (Lima, OH: Wyndham Hall Press).

Morgan, John H. (2018). *The Learning Spectrum in Child Development: Developmental Psychology in Maria Montessori, Jean Piaget, and Erik Erikson* (Levering, MI: Wyndham Hall Press).

Morgan, John H. (2020). *Sigmund Freud Comprehensive Reference Dictionary of Psychoanalysis* (Levering, MI: Wyndham Hall Press).

Mullahy, P. (1970). *Psychoanalysis and Interpersonal Psychiatry: The Contributions of Harry Stack Sullivan.* N.Y.: Science House.

Nausheen B, Gidron Y, Peveler R, Moss-Morris R. "Social support and cancer progression: a systematic review". *Journal of Psychosomatic Research.* 2009: 67 (5): 403–15.

Noll, Richard (2011). *American Madness: The Rise and Fall of Dementia Praecox.* Cambridge and London: Harvard University Press.

Osborn RL, Demoncada AC, Feuerstein M . "Psychosocial interventions for depression, anxiety, and quality of life in cancer survivors: meta-analyses". *International Journal of Psychiatry in Medicine. 2006:* 36 (1): 13–34.

Park CL, Edmondson D, Fenster JR, Blank TO. "Meaning making and psychological adjustment following cancer: the mediating roles of growth, life meaning, and restored just-world beliefs". *Journal of Consulting and Clinical Psychology.* 2008: 76 (5): 863–75.

Patel, S.B., McCall, W.V. "Interface of Psychiatric Services with Urological Oncology Practice." *European Urology Focus. 2020:* 05 May, 6(6):1140-1141.

Perry, H. S. (1982). *Psychiatrist of America: The Life of Harry Stack Sullivan.* London: The Belknap Press of Harvard University Press.

Petticrew M, Bell R, Hunter D. "Influence of psychological coping on survival and recurrence in people with cancer:

systematic review". *BMJ (Clinical Research Ed.)*. 2002: 325 (7372): 1066.

Phelps, A.C., Lauderdale, K.E., Alcorn, S., Dillinger, J., Balboni, M.T., Van Wert, M., VanderWeele, T.J., and Balboni, T.A. Addressing spirituality within the care of patients at the end of life: perspectives of advanced cancer patients, oncologists, and oncology nurses. *Journal of Clinical Oncology*, 2012: 30:2538-2544.

Quante, Aim, Schulz, Kristina, Fissler, Maria. "Psychiatric Comorbidities in Cancer Patients: Acute Interventons by the Psychiatric Consultation Liaison Service." *Wien Med. Worchenschr 2020:* Oct; 170 (13-14): 348-356.

Reber, Arthur S. (1985). *The Penguin Dictionary of Psychology* (London: Viking Press).

Riba, Michelle and Luigi Grassi. (2012). *Clinical Psycho-Oncology: An International Perspective* (London: John Wiley and Sons).

Rapp SR, Vrana S. "Substituting nonsomatic for somatic symptoms in the diagnosis of depression in elderly male medical patients." *Am J Psychiatry.* 1989;146:1197–2000.

Rodin, D., Balboni M., Mitchell, C., Smith, P.T., VanderWeele, T.J., and Balboni, T.A. Whose role? Oncology practitioners' perceptions of their role in providing spiritual care to advanced cancer patients. *Supportive Care and Cancer*, 2015: 23:2543-2550.

Rogers, Carl R. (1970). *On Becoming a Person: A Therapist's View of Psychotherapy* (Boston: Houghton Mifflin Company.

Rouleau CR, Garland SN, Carlson LE. "The impact of mindfulness-based interventions on symptom burden, positive psychological outcomes, and biomarkers in cancer patients". *Cancer Management and Research.* 2015: 7: 121–31.

Roth S, Cohen LJ. "Approach, avoidance, and coping with stress". *The American Psychologist. 1986:* 41 (7): 813–9.

Sajatovic, M., Sanders, R., Alexeenko, L., Madhusoodanan, S. "Primary Prevention of Psychiatric Illness in Special Populations." *Annals of Clinical Psychiatry. 2010:* Nov; 22(4): 262-273.

Schultz, Duane P. and Sydney Ellen Schultz (6th Edition). (1996). *A History of Modern Psychology* (New York: Harcourt Brace College Publishers).

Shepherd, M. "Two faces of Emil Kraepelin". *The British Journal of Psychiatry.* 1995: 167 (2): 174–183.

Shimizu K, Akizuki N, Nakaya N, Fujimori M, Fujisawa D, Ogawa A, et al. "Treatment response to psychiatric intervention and predictors of response among cancer patients with adjustment disorders." *J Pain Symptom Manage.* 2011;41:684–91.

Shorter, Edward. (1997). *A History of Psychiatry: From the Era of the Asylum to the Age of Prozac* (N.Y.: John Wiley & Sons).

Simpson, Scott A., Chwastiak, Lydia A., Andrews, Sarah R., Bienvenu, O. Joseph et. al. "Updates in Consultation-Liaison Psychiatry." *Psychosomatics.* 2020: Sept-Oct; 61 (5): 450-455.

Sperner-Unterweger, B. "Psycho-oncology – Psychosocial oncology: Integration in a Concpet of Oncological Treatment." *Nervenarzt.* 2011: March; 82 (3): 371-378.

Stanton AL, Danoff-Burg S, Sworowski LA, Collins CA, Branstetter AD, Rodriguez-Hanley A, et al. "Randomized, controlled trial of written emotional expression and benefit finding in breast cancer patients". *Journal of Clinical Oncology*. 2002: 20 (20): 4160–8.

Subnis UB, Farb NA, Piedalue KL, Speca M, Lupichuk S, Tang PA, et al. "A Smartphone App-Based Mindfulness Intervention for Cancer Survivors: Protocol for a Randomized Controlled Trial". *JMIR Research Protocols*. 2020: 9 (5): e15178.

Sullivan, Harry Stack (1953). *Conceptions of Modern Psychiatry: The First William Alanson White Memorial Lectures*, NY: W. W. Norton & Co.

Sullivan, Harry Stack (1965). *Personal Psychopathology*, NY: W. W. Norton & Co.

Sullivan, Harry Stack (1953). *The Interpersonal Theory of Psychiatry*, NY: W. W. Norton & Co.

Sullivan, Harry Stack (1954). *The Psychiatric Interview*, NY: W. W. Norton & Co.

Sullivan, Harry Stack (1956). *Clinical Studies in Psychiatry*, NY: W. W. Norton & Co.

Sullivan, Harry Stack (1962). *Schizophrenia as a Human Process*, NY: W. W. Norton & Co.

Sullivan, Harry Stack (1964). *The Fusion of Psychiatry and Social Science*, NY: W. W. Norton & Co.

Syrjala KL, Jensen MP, Mendoza ME, Yi JC, Fisher HM, Keefe FJ. "Psychological and behavioral approaches to cancer pain management". *Journal of Clinical Oncology*. 2014: 32 (16): 1703–11.

Vallurupalli, M., Lauderdale, K., Balboni, M.J., Prigerson, H.G., Phelps, A.C., VanderWeele, T.J., and Balboni, T.A. The role of spirituality and religious coping in the quality of life of patients receiving palliative radiation therapy. *Journal of Supportive Oncology*, 2012: 10:81-87.

Valtorta NK, Kanaan M, Gilbody S, Ronzi S, Hanratty B. "Loneliness and social isolation as risk factors for coronary heart disease and stroke: systematic review and meta-analysis of longitudinal observational studies". *Heart (British Cardiac Society)*. 2016: 102 (13): 1009–16.

Waldron EA, Janke EA, Bechtel CF, Ramirez M, Cohen A. "A systematic review of psychosocial interventions to improve cancer caregiver quality of life". *Psycho-oncology*. 2013: 22 (6): 1200–7.

Watson, Maggie, Dunn, Jeff, Holland, Jimmie C. "Review of the History and Development in the field of Psychosocial Oncology." *International Review of Psychiatry 2014:* Feb; 26 (1): 128-135.

Westermair, A.L., Schreiber, W., Dumchen, J., Perrar, K. M. "Psychiatrists in Palliative Care of People with Severe Psychiatric Illnesses and an Oncological Comorbidity." *Nervenarzt 2020* May; 91 (5): 404-410.

Winkelman, W.D., Lauderdale, K., Balboni, M.J., Phelps, A.C., Block, S.D., VanderWeele, T.J., and Balboni, T.A. The relationship of spiritual concerns to the quality of life of advanced cancer patients. *Journal of Palliative Medicine*, 2011: 14:1022-1028.

Wood, Debra (2004). "It Begins with an RN: Pearl Moore, ONS CEO". *NurseZone.*

Zabora J, BrintzenhofeSzoc K, Curbow B, Hooker C, Piantadosi S. "The prevalence of psychological distress by cancer site". *Psycho-oncology. 2001:* 10 (1): 19–28.

Zainal NZ, Booth S, Huppert FA. "The efficacy of mindfulness-based stress reduction on mental health of breast cancer patients: a meta-analysis". Psycho-Oncology. 2013: 22 (7): 1457–65.

Zeig, Jeffrey K., Editor (1987). *The Evolution of Psychotherapy* (New York: Brunner/Mazel Publishers).

Zeng Y, Luo T, Xie H, Huang M, Cheng AS. "Health benefits of qigong or tai chi for cancer patients: a systematic review and meta-analyses". Complementary Therapies in Medicine. 2014: 22 (1): 173–86.

Zepstein-Peterson, Z.D., Sullivan, A.J., Enzinger, A.C., Trevino, K.M., Zollfrank, A.A., Balboni, M.J., VanderWeele, T.J., Balboni, T.A. Examining forms of spiritual care provided in the advanced cancer setting. *American Journal of Hospice and Palliative Medicine*, 2015: 23:2543-2550.

Zielazny, P., Zielinska, P., de Walden-Galuszko, K., Kuziemski, K., Bethowska-Korpala, B. "Psychooncology in Poland." *Psychiatr. Pol. 2016:* Oct 31: 50(5): 1065-1073.

Zigmond AS, Snaith RP. "The Hospital anxiety and Depression Scale." *Acta Psychiatr Scand.* 1983;67:361–70.

Zollfrank, A.A., Trevino, K.M., Cadge, W., Balboni, M.J., Thiel, M.M., Fitchett, G., Gallivan, K., VanderWeele, T.J., and Balboni, T.A. Teaching healthcare providers to provide spiritual care: a pilot study. *Journal of Palliative Medicine*, 2015: 18:408-414.

Zolnierek KB, Dimatteo MR. "Physician communication and patient adherence to treatment: a meta-analysis". *Medical Care.* 2009: 47 (8): 826–34.

Books by John H. Morgan

from Wyndham Hall Press/Amazon Books

- *Schizophrenia: The Enduring Challenge to Psychiatric Practice*
- *A Summary Guide to the Collected Works of Sigmund Freud*
- *Sigmund Freud Comprehensive Reference Dictionary of Psychoanalysis*
- *Harry Stack Sullivan Encyclopedic Dictionary of Interpersonal Psychotherapy*
- *Psychopathology: A Clinical Guide to Personality Disorders*
- *Clinical Psychotherapy: A History of Theory and Practice*
- *Understanding Ourselves: Essays in the History & Philosophy of the Social Sciences*
- *Child Psychopathology in Clinical Practice: The Psychoanalytic Theories of Karen Horney, Melanie Klein, and Anna Freud*
- *The Learning Spectrum in Child Development: Developmental Psychology in Maria Montessori, Jean Piaget, and Erik Erikson*

- *Geriatric Psychotherapy: Essays in Clinical Practice and Counseling Psychology*
- *The Scope of Modern Psychiatry: Treatment Options in Clinical Practice*
- *The Damaged Self: Exploring the Psychopathology of a Diminished Life*
- *The Morgan Reader: A Compendium of Scholarly Papers*

ABOUT THE AUTHOR

John Henry Morgan, Ph.D.(Hartford), D.Sc.(London), Psy.D.(FH/Oxford), Senior Fellow in Behavioral Science *emeritus,* Foundation House/Oxford (UK), was educated at Harvard, Yale, and Princeton in the behavioral sciences from which he held six postdoctoral research appointments. Dr. Morgan recently retired from teaching a doctoral-level seminar for 20 years in the International Summer Program of Oxford University during which time he also served concurrently as a Postdoctoral Visiting Scholar at New York University as well as holding an appointment as Postdoctoral Research Scholar at the University of Chicago. Prior to his years of teaching at Oxford University, he held an appointment as the National Science Foundation Science Faculty Fellow at the University of Notre Dame.